SMALL ANIMAL NEUROANATOMIC
LESION LOCALIZATION PRACTICE BOOK

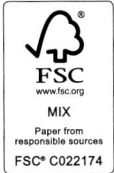

SMALL ANIMAL NEUROANATOMIC LESION LOCALIZATION PRACTICE BOOK

Edited by

Heidi Barnes Heller

*Barnes Veterinary Specialty Services,
Madison, Wisconsin, USA*

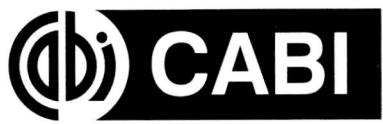

CABI is a trading name of CAB International

CABI	CABI
Nosworthy Way	200 Portland Street
Wallingford	Boston
Oxfordshire OX10 8DE	MA 02114
UK	USA
Tel: +44 (0)1491 832111	Tel: +1 (617)682-9015
E-mail: info@cabi.org	E-mail: cabi-nao@cabi.org
Website: www.cabi.org	

A catalogue record for this book is available from the British Library, London, UK.

ISBN-13: 9781789247923 (paperback)
            9781789247930 (ePDF)
            9781789247947 (ePub)

DOI: 10.1079/9781789247947.0000

Commissioning Editor: Alexandra Lainsbury
Editorial Assistant: Emma McCann
Production Editor: Marta Patiño

Typeset by SPi, Pondicherry, India
Printed and bound in the UK by Severn, Gloucester

Contents

Contributors

Susan Arnold, DVM, DACVIM (Neurology), Department of Veterinary Clinical Sciences, Lewis Small Animal Hospital, University of Minnesota College of Veterinary Medicine, 1352 Boyd Avenue, C310, St. Paul, MN 55108, USA. Email: saarnold@umn.edu

Heidi Barnes Heller, DVM, DACVIM (Neurology), Barnes Veterinary Specialty Services, 2226 County Road F, Barneveld, WI 53507 (Madison), USA. Email: barnes@barnesveterinaryservices.com

Joy Delamaide Gasper, DVM, DACVIM (Neurology), Department of Neurology, Madison Veterinary Specialists, 2704 Royal Avenue, Madison, WI 53713, USA. Email: JDelamaide@mvsvets.com

Kari Foss, DVM, DACVIM (Neurology), Department of Veterinary Clinical Medicine, University of Illinois College of Veterinary Medicine, 2001 S. Lincoln Avenue, Urbana, IL 61802, USA, Email: karifoss@illinois.edu

Julien Guevar, DVM, MVM, DECVN, MRCVS, Vetsuisse Faculty, University of Bern, Langgassstrasse 120, 3012 Bern, Switzerland. Email: julien.guevar@vetsuisse.unibe.ch

Devon Hague, DVM, ACVIM (Neurology), Department of Veterinary Clinical Medicine, Veterinary Teaching Hospital University of Illinois, 2001 S. Lincoln Avenue, Urbana, IL 61802, USA. Email: hague@illinois.edu

Sam Long, BVSc, PhD, DECVN, Veterinary Referral Hospital, 36 Lonsdale Street, Dandenong, Victoria 3175, Australia. Email: sam.long@vrh247.com.au

Simon Platt, BVM&S, DACVIM (Neurology), FRCVS, ECVN, Veterinary Neurology Training LLC, Watkinsville, GA, 30677, USA. Email: srplatt1@gmail.com

Helena Rylander, DVM, DACVIM (Neurology), University of Wisconsin–Madison, 2015 Linden Drive, Madison, WI 53706, USA. Email: Helena.rylander@wisc.edu

Abbreviations

AChR	acetylcholine receptor
ACTH	adrenocorticotropic hormone
ALT	alanine aminotransferase
ANNPE	acute, noncompressive nucleus pulposus extrusion
APN	acute polyradiculoneuropathy
AST	aspartate aminotransferase
AU	both ears
BAER	brainstem auditory evoked response
BAR	bright, alert, responsive
BCS	body condition score
CBC	complete blood count
CK	creatine kinase
CMAP	compound muscle action potential
CN I–XII	cranial nerves I–XII
CNS	central nervous system
CPK	creatine phosphokinase
CRD	complex repetitive discharge
CRIDP	chronic (relapsing) inflammatory demyelinating polyneuropathy
CRT	capillary refill time
CSF	cerebrospinal fluid
CT	computed tomography
CVA	cerebrovascular accident
DAMNITV	degenerative, anomalous, metabolic, neoplastic, nutritional, inflammatory, idiopathic, toxic, traumatic, vascular (classification of diseases)
DMD	Duchenne muscular dystrophy
ECG	electrocardiogram

EENT	eyes, ears, nose, and throat
EMG	electromyography
FCEM	fibrocartilaginous embolic myelopathy
FIP	feline infectious peritonitis
FLAIR	fluid-attenuated inversion recovery
GI	gastrointestinal
GME	granulomatous meningoencephalitis
GRMD	Golden Retriever muscular dystrophy
hpf	high power field
IgG	immunoglobulin G
IgM	immunoglobulin M
IV	intravenous
LMN	lower motor neuron
MRI	magnetic resonance imaging
MUO	meningoencephalitis of unknown origin
NALL	neuroanatomic lesion localization
NLE	necrotizing leukoencephalitis
NME	necrotizing meningoencephalitis
NSAID	nonsteroidal anti-inflammatory drug
OD	right eye
OS	left eye
OU	both eyes
P	pulse
$PaCO_2$	partial pressure of carbon dioxide
PaO_2	partial pressure of oxygen
PCR	polymerase chain reaction
PLR	pupillary light reflex
PMMA	polymethylmethacrylate
PNS	peripheral nervous system
PO	per os (given orally)
q8h	every 8 h
q8–12h	every 8–12 h
q12h	every 12 h
q24h	every 24 h
QAR	quiet, alert, responsive
R	respiration
RAS	reticular activating system
RBC	red blood cell
SNAP 4Dx Plus	a rapid screening test for indicating infection with selected common canine vector-borne agents (heartworm, Lyme, *Ehrlichia canis*, *Ehrlichia ewingi*, *Anaplasma phagocytophilum*, and *Anaplasma platys*)
STIR	short tau inversion recovery
T	temperature
T1W	T1-weighted
T2W	T2-weighted

T2*W	T2*-weighted
T4	thyroxine
TNCC	total nucleated cell count
TSH	thyroid-stimulating hormone
UMN	upper motor neuron
USG	urine specific gravity
WBC	white blood cell

1 How to Use this Book

HEIDI BARNES HELLER*

Barnes Veterinary Specialty Services, Madison, Wisconsin, USA

The purpose of this book is to help you sharpen your small animal NALL skills. It is assumed that you have progressed through your neuroanatomy courses in school and are either in clinics, internship, residency, or in clinical practice. This is not a neuroanatomy book but there may be discussion pertaining to neuroanatomy in the following cases. If you're unsure of the neuroanatomy being discussed, please refer to a veterinary neuroanatomy text for a more de-tailed anatomic discussion (Chrisman *et al.*, 2002; de Lahunta and Glass, 2009; Dewey and da Costa, 2015). The focus of this book is to practice NALL. The chapters contain cases that will facilitate this practice. Case practice is the key to improving NALL skills.

Within each case you will find the following headings:

- Patient signalment;
- History;
- Physical examination;
- Neurologic examination;
- Neuroanatomic lesion localization practice sheet;
- Discussion on neuroanatomic lesion localization;
- Neuroanatomic lesion localization;
- Differential diagnoses;
- Diagnostic testing and results; and
- Case conclusion.

Please read the chapter about performing the neurologic examination. By reading this chapter first it will be clear what has been included in the neurologic

*Email: barnes@barnesveterinaryservices.com

DOI: 10.1079/9781789247947.0001

examination when a clinician lists the findings as "all normal". This chapter may also be a good resource when performing the neurologic examination with live patients within your own practice. You may wish to design your own checklist to ensure you include each portion of the exam, every time.

After you have read the neurologic examination, you are encouraged to complete the neuroanatomic lesion localization practice sheet included in the chapter before progressing to the discussion on neuroanatomic lesion localization table provided in the case. Extra practice sheets are provided in the Appendix at the end of this book. Remember: Practice, practice, practice!

How to Use the Practice Sheet

When an abnormality is identified in the neurologic examination, write the abnormality in the form in the far-left column, similar to the way "head tilt" is written below.

Abnormality	Possible NALL	Possible NALL	Possible NALL
Head tilt			

After adding the abnormality on the form, list all possible NALL for this abnormality. For the listed abnormality, "head tilt", add the following NALL that may cause the signs noted. Importantly, do not eliminate a NALL based on other case information provided.

Abnormality	Possible NALL	Possible NALL	Possible NALL
Head tilt	Peripheral CN VIII	Brainstem/medulla	Cerebellum

Repeat this task for all of the reported abnormalities in the case. After you finish listing the abnormalities and the possible NALL, review the possible NALL and eliminate those that do not apply based on other information in the case. For help understanding the neurologic examination and NALL, please see Chapter 2. Below, the remaining abnormalities in our imaginary case example have been added.

Abnormality	Possible NALL	Possible NALL	Possible NALL
Head tilt	Peripheral CN VIII	Brainstem/medulla	Cerebellum
Nystagmus	Peripheral CN VIII		
Hypermetria	Cerebellum		

At the conclusion of this step, you will see an opportunity to stop and determine the NALL before proceeding to the author's summary of the NALL, differential diagnoses, diagnostic testing and results, and case conclusion. Additional assistance with NALL may be found using reference texts listed at the end of this chapter (Chrisman *et al.*, 2002; de Lahunta and Glass, 2009; Dewey and da Costa, 2015).

Abnormality	Possible NALL	Possible NALL	Possible NALL
Head tilt	~~Peripheral CN VIII~~	~~Brainstem/medulla~~	Cerebellum
Nystagmus	~~Peripheral CN VIII~~	~~Brainstem/medulla~~	Cerebellum
Hypermetria	Cerebellum		

In this imaginary case, the only scenario in which all three findings can associate together is if the NALL is in the cerebellum; therefore the NALL for this example case is the cerebellum. Check your answers against those of the author and then proceed to the case summary and conclusion. More practice sheets are available in the Appendix at the end of this book for additional practice.

Unless otherwise noted, all images and videos are owned by the lead author.

References

Chrisman, C.L., Mariani, C., Platt, S. and Clemmons, R. (2002) *Neurology for the Small Animal Practitioner (Made Easy Series)*, 1st edn. Teton NewMedia, New York.
de Lahunta, A. and Glass, E. (2009) *Veterinary Neuroanatomy and Clinical Neurology*, 3rd edn. Saunders Elsevier, St. Louis, Missouri.
Dewey, C.W. and da Costa, R.C. (2015) *Practical Guide to Canine and Feline Neurology*, 3rd edn. Wiley, Hoboken, New Jersey.

2 Introduction to the Neurologic Examination

Heidi Barnes Heller*

Barnes Veterinary Specialty Services, Madison, Wisconsin, USA

Unless otherwise noted, all images and videos are owned by the lead author.

Anatomic and Functional Organization of the Nervous System

The nervous system is divided into the CNS and the PNS. The CNS is composed of the brain and spinal cord. The PNS is composed of the peripheral nerves, neuromuscular junction, and muscles.

Brain refers to all neurologic tissue within the cranial vault (Table 2.1). We often combine parts of the CNS together in conversation to denote sections of the nervous system that commonly present with similar signs. You should also be familiar with the terms prosencephalon (inclusive of cerebrum, thalamus, and thalamic components) and brainstem (inclusive of midbrain, pons, and medulla oblongata) (Fig. 2.1).

The difference between function and anatomic organization of the nervous system, especially as it relates to the thalamus and some of the tracts, can be confusing. In clinical neurology, functional organization, not anatomic organization, is used for NALL. This means that the functional brainstem is composed of mesencephalon, metencephalon, and myelencephalon (Table 2.2).

Patient Signalment, History, Physical Examination

1. Signalment.
   - Species: There are diseases that are more common in certain species.
   - Breed: Some diseases are more common in specific breeds. It is important to note that this does not exclude mixed-breed dogs and domestic cats from developing diseases common to a specific breed.

---

*Email: barnes@barnesveterinaryservices.com

© CAB International 2022. *Small Animal Neuroanatomic Lesion Localization Practice Book*
(ed. H. Barnes Heller)
DOI: 10.1079/9781789247947.0002

Table 2.1. English definitions, followed by the definition, for common anatomic divisions in the brain.

English term	Definition
Brain	All neurologic tissue within the cranial vault
Forebrain	Refers to the prosencephalon (cerebrum, thalamus, thalamic components)
Hindbrain	Metencephalon (pons) and myelencephalon (medulla)
Brainstem	Midbrain, pons, and medulla oblongata

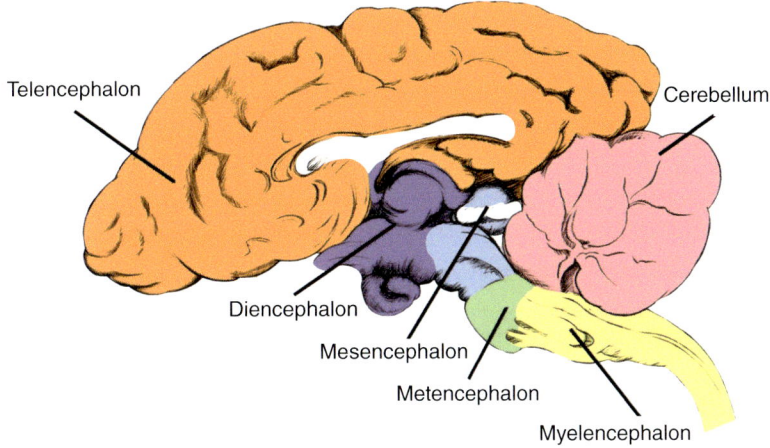

Fig. 2.1. Lateral view of the intracranial structures including forebrain, brainstem, and cerebellum. (Image used with permission from Dr. Pam Boutilier.)

Table 2.2. The intracranial components of the brain may be described in their Latin or English terminology.

Latin term	English term
Telencephalon	Cerebrum
Diencephalon	Thalamus, hypothalamus, epithalamus, and subthalamus
Mesencephalon	Midbrain
Metencephalon	Pons
Myelencephalon	Medulla oblongata
Cerebellum	Cerebellum

- Age: Congenital disorders present in younger patients and neoplasia and degenerative disorders are more common in older patients.

2. History.
- The type of onset (peracute, acute, chronic, or waxing/waning) and progression (progression versus nonprogressive) classification of clinical signs are important when formulating a differential diagnoses list but is not critical for NALL.

- Progression:
  - ○ Acute nonprogressive signs suggest vascular accident (i.e., infarct, hemorrhage) or trauma.
  - ○ Acute progressive signs suggest inflammatory/infectious disease.
  - ○ Chronic, progressive signs suggest degenerative diseases or neoplasia.
  - ○ Static nonprogressive signs suggest developmental diseases or prior injury.
3. Physical examination.
  - This is performed to identify comorbidities, or copy-cat diseases. Copy-cat diseases are conditions that may exhibit signs similar to a neurologic disease but when you look closely, the disease isn't affecting the neurologic system. Examples of copy-cat diseases are bilateral cruciate ligament rupture giving the appearance of UMN paraparesis, and syncopal collapse appearing like a seizure.

Neurologic Examination

A complete neurologic examination must include all of the following components of the exam. If you have a digital record-keeping system, writing each of the components in a digital form may assist with record keeping.

Observation of mentation

Initial observations of a pet in the exam space can provide insight into their level of mentation. The author prefers these common terms used to describe the mentation of dogs and cats; however other terms are used in the literature:

- Normal: BAR or QAR.
- Obtunded: Lethargic and less responsive to the environment. The degree of obtunded may be graded mild, moderate, or severe in condition. Although somewhat subjective, mildly obtunded suggests a response is present to auditory, tactile, and visual stimulation but that the response is delayed or muted from normal. A moderate level of obtundation suggests a response to auditory or tactile only and severe obtundation suggests that only a response to tactile stimuli remains.
- Coma: Unconscious and unresponsive to painful stimulus with only reflex activity present.

Gait and body posture

Body posture refers to the position of the body in reference to normal. Terms such as head tilt, head turn, or opisthotonos may be used to describe body posture. The head tilt suggests vestibular dysfunction; head or body turn suggests disease of the forebrain/prosencephalon; decerebellate rigidity is suggestive of a lesion in the cerebellar peduncles or cerebellum, and includes opisthotonos (dorsiflexion of the head and the neck), extensor rigidity in the thoracic limbs, and flexed or extended pelvic limbs with alert mentation. Decerebrate rigidity is suggestive of a lesion in the midbrain or pons. Signs include opisthotonos, extensor rigidity of all four limbs and the trunk, and decreased mentation (i.e., coma); and finally Schiff-Sherrington posture is associated with an acute, severe spinal injury between T2 and L4 spinal cord segments (de Lahunta and Glass, 2009). Signs include increased tone in the thoracic limbs with flaccid paralysis of the pelvic limbs when recumbent.

Gait is described as ataxia, paresis, or lameness. There are three types of ataxia:

- Proprioceptive ataxia is an indication of a spinal cord, brainstem, or fore-brain disease. Ataxia is not noted with neuromuscular disease. Signs of proprioceptive ataxia include a crossing of the limbs when walking down a straight pathway, or placing the limbs narrow and wide of the midline of the body without consistency.
- Vestibular ataxia indicates dysfunction of the vestibular apparatus. When observing a patient with vestibular ataxia, the observer can appreciate a falling or drifting toward one side when walking. This can be especially magnified when the patient is turned in a circle.
- Cerebellar ataxia occurs with disease or injury to the cerebellum. Signs of hypermetria, truncal sway, and a wide-based stance with or without intention tremor are indications of cerebellar ataxia. The hypermetria is ipsilateral to the lesion and can, therefore, be useful for NALL.

Paresis is a weak movement or incomplete paralysis. This involves most commonly UMNs or LMNs, but remember the neuromuscular junction, muscle and bones, or joints can be a source of paresis also. A patient with mild paresis will exhibit a reduced joint range of motion when walking, giving the appearance of shuffling. Severe paresis may be more profound so that an animal is unable to support weight even with purposeful limb movements. Paresis may be further described according to the leg or legs affected (Table 2.3).

Table 2.3. Descriptive terminology used for more specific classification of paresis.

Term	Definition
Ambulatory	Able to support own body weight and move purposefully
Para-	Pelvic legs
Tetra-	All four legs
Hemi-	One half (left or right)
-plegia	Unable to move legs AT ALL. Motor function can be assessed by walking away and calling the patient, or by supporting the patient under the pelvis and the chest and encouraging the patient to move forward. Avoid carrying by tail
-paresis	Weak but able to move legs, on own, with or without support
Ataxia	Wobbly—i.e., failure of muscle coordination
Lameness	A change in stride length, or character. May be orthopedic or neurologic in origin

Finally, lameness is noted as inappropriate weight bearing during the standing or, less commonly, swinging phase of the gait. Although commonly orthopedic, neurologic lameness may occur with nerve root impingement or inflammation. Neurologic lameness may be termed a root signature sign.

Cranial nerve examination

Evaluation of the 12 paired cranial nerves provides insight into the function of the brainstem and forebrain. Detailed description of the technique for examining these nerves can be found elsewhere (Rylander, 2013), and will be reviewed in brief below. It is important to understand how to perform the evaluation, as well as be able to associate the cranial nerve with its functional brainstem segment (Table 2.4).

The functional brainstem segment is where the cell body is, or is mostly, contained. The olfactory nerve is the exception because this grouping of nerves is associated with the olfactory bulb of the forebrain. Although optic nerve cell bodies are in the thalamus, dysfunction is attributed commonly to dysfunction of both the thalamus and the cerebrum (forebrain).

- Olfactory nerve is usually not tested because it is difficult to clinically evaluate.
- Menace response: Menace response is best learned by manually drawing out the pathway when evaluating a patient with a menace deficit. Functional CN II is treated as a crossing track in dogs and cats unless it is being outlined for vision. If a menacing hand gesture is made in front of the animal's face, the visual stimuli are transmitted along CN II, crossing at the chiasm, and traced to the opposite cerebrum. To blink, a large, multistep reflex pathway is activated which starts in the cerebrum and ends with synapse on the nucleus of CN VII at the level of the medulla oblongata. At this point, the animal will blink its eye. Dysfunction of CN II, opposite cerebrum, and ipsilateral CN VII can cause a menace response deficit. PLR testing is employed to evaluate CN II separately from CN VII and the cerebrum. Menace response involves CN II, opposite prosencephalon, or CN VII. If the menace response is absent, dropping a cotton ball in front of either eye watching for a response can help assess vision.
- PLR: For PLR testing, light is shone into the eye and transmitted down the same CN II. Prior to entering the prosencephalon, for the menace response, it dives into the midbrain to synapse on the parasympathetic nucleus of CN III. Parasympathetic fibers then pass along CN III back to the eye to constrict the pupil. Damage to CN II, midbrain, or CN III can result in PLR deficits.
- Strabismus means an abnormal position of the eye. This can be at rest or with movement. CN III, CN IV, and CN VI must be abnormal if an animal is exhibiting a resting strabismus. A handy mnemonic to help remember what cranial nerve innervates what muscle is: LR6 SO4 AO3, LR = lateral rectus muscle; SO = superior (dorsal) oblique; AO = all other muscles.

Table 2.4. The cranial nerves and examination performed during the neurologic examination.

CN	Name	Functional anatomic localization	What does it do?	How do you test it?
I	Olfactory	Cerebrum	Sense of smell	Observation
II	Optic	Thalamus	Sense of vision	Menace, visual testing, PLR
III	Oculomotor	Midbrain	Somatic movement to the eye and carries parasympathetic fibers for PLR	Evaluation for strabismus, physiologic nystagmus, and PLR
IV	Trochlear	Midbrain	Motor to periocular muscles	Evaluation of physiologic nystagmus and strabismus
V	Trigeminal	Pons	Sensory to face, cornea. Motor to muscles of mastication	Corneal, blink reflex, open jaw for tone
VI	Abducent	Medulla	Motor to periocular muscles	Strabismus/eye movement
VII	Facial	Medulla	Motor to facial muscles	Blink, auricular reflex, and lip twitch
VIII	Vestibulocochlear	Medulla	Hearing and balance	Observation, physiologic nystagmus, positional strabismus
IX	Glossopharyngeal	Medulla	Sensory to pharynx	Sensory for gag reflex
X	Vagus	Medulla	Motor to pharynx, heart rate, GI motility	Motor for gag reflex
XI	Spinal accessory	Medulla	Motor to trapezius, sternocephalicus, and brachiocephalicus muscles	Palpation for symmetry
XII	Hypoglossal	Medulla	Motor to tongue	Observation

Animals with damage to CN III will have a ventrolateral strabismus. Damage to CN IV causes a rotational strabismus and damage to CN VI causes a medial strabismus. Strabismus is noted when the animal is at rest, NOT when you move the head. A movement-induced strabismus is called a positional strabismus and is noted with damage to CN VIII only.

- Oculocephalic reflex (physiologic nystagmus) assesses how well CN VIII coordinates CN III, CN IV, and CN VI as the head is moved. As the head is moved slowly from side to side, the eyes should flick following the direction of the head movement. Inappropriate physiologic nystagmus typically indicates damage to CN VIII most commonly.

- Palpebral reflex: Stimulation of the medial canthus (ophthalmic branch of CN V) and the lateral canthus (maxillary branch of CN V) should result in a blink of the eyelids activated by CN VII. The maxillary branch of CN V is tested by touching the nasal mucosa or the upper lip (vibrissae) and the mandibular branch is tested by touching the mandibular fur. The response that is desired is movement of the facial muscles (CN VII) and/or movement of the head (conscious response from the cerebrum).
- The auricular reflex has a sensory and motor component both performed by CN VII. A gentle stimulus is applied to the rostral pinna which should result in an ear flick.
- Symmetry of face: The facial nerve is the motor pathway to the muscles of facial expression. Asymmetry of the face indicates a CN VII problem.
- Palpation of temporalis and masticatory muscles: The motor branch of the mandibular branch of the trigeminal nerve (CN V) innervates the masticatory muscles. Masticatory muscle atrophy indicates a lesion in this branch of CN V or of the muscle itself (i.e., myopathy).
- Corneal reflex: The cornea is innervated by the ophthalmic branch of CN V, and the retractor bulbi muscle is innervated by CN VI. When the cornea is gently touched, the globe should retract. Assessing CN V usually results in motor activation of CN VII; however the corneal reflex allows the practitioner to isolate the sensory action of CN V from the motor activity of CN VII, by employing motor activity of CN VI instead.
- Spontaneous (or resting) nystagmus indicates a problem with CN VIII. Hearing is not routinely evaluated during examination but could be evaluated using a BAER.
- Gag reflex: The gag reflex is formed by stimulation of the glossopharyngeal nerve through direct stimulation of the oropharynx and observing a muscle constriction that results in a "gag" sound or the feeling of constriction around the practitioner's fingers. An internal gag reflex is performed by placing one or two fingers in the oropharynx and observing constriction sounds and motion. An external gag reflex can be performed by rapidly constricting the oropharynx proximal to the larynx and observing for the same sound or movement. For animals in which vaccine status is unknown, or if the animal is aggressive, external gag should be performed.
- Palpation of the neck for symmetry: The accessory nerve (CN XI) innervates the trapezius, sternocephalicus, and brachiocephalicus muscles. A lesion affecting only this nerve is difficult to recognize but may result in atrophy of the neck muscles.
- Tongue tone, tongue symmetry, and tongue movement are observed by opening the animal's mouth and visualizing the tongue at rest and at movement. Abnormal innervation of CN XII (hypoglossal nerve) may result in muscle atrophy and restricted movement. Note that a tongue protruding from the mouth is normal for some breeds or may be related to a loss of dentition. This should not be mistaken for damage to CN XII.

Evaluation of postural reaction

Postural reaction, most commonly includes the following tests. Detailed description of the neuroanatomy involved with these tests can be found in other sources (de Lahunta and Glass, 2009):

- Paw replacement test: While providing support, and on stable footing such as a yoga mat or rug, turn a paw over and place it on the dorsum of the paw. The animal should right the paw to the normal position with minimal to no delay or scuffing (Fig. 2.2).
- Placing (visual or tactile): This is a useful test for cats! The animal is blinded and advanced toward a horizontal surface such that the paw gently touches the surface. A correct response occurs when the animal lifts the limb. They may try to place the limb on the surface; however this is not required.
- Hopping: With one leg on the ground, the other three legs are lifted carefully by the examiner. While ensuring the animal does not fall, they are pushed laterally on the leg that remained on the ground. A proper response is a hopping motion on the limb. Remember: The animal is expected to hop, the practitioner is not expected to hop the animal on the limb.

Postural reaction abnormalities indicate a neurologic problem. The pathway for all postural reaction testing is peripheral nerve → ipsilateral spinal cord → ipsilateral medulla and pons → cross in midbrain → end in prosencephalon. Some branches also: peripheral nerve → ipsilateral spinal cord → ipsilateral medulla → ipsilateral cerebellum. It is important to utilize the remainder of the neurologic examination to help you localize the lesion.

Evaluation of spinal reflexes

Examination of the spinal reflexes tests the integrity of the sensory and motor components of the reflex arch and the soundness of descending motor pathways, as appropriate, on the reflex arch. The pleximeter is used to hit on the

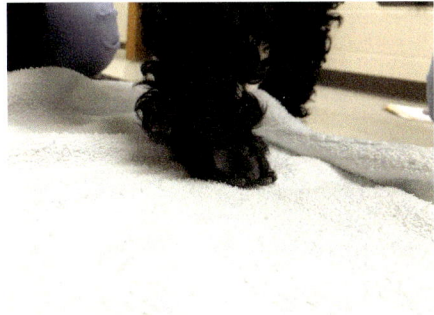

Fig. 2.2. An example of a dog with a paw replacement deficit demonstrating the dorsal positioning of the paw that is needed to perform this postural reaction.

tendon to the muscle tested, or at times on the user's finger. Repositioning of the limb to obtain the reflex may be needed multiple times; keep trying.

An absent or decreased reflex indicates partial or complete loss of the sensory or motor components of the reflex. Reduced or absent reflexes in the thoracic limbs indicate a lesion in the C6–T2 spinal cord segment and reduced or absent reflexes in the pelvic limbs indicate a lesion in the L4–S3 spinal cord segments. Reduced reflexes in all limbs may indicate a multifocal myelopathy or a nonspinal NALL.

An exaggerated reflex is rarely clinically useful because visualizing something in motion to be "more" than normal motion is rarely reliable. Factors that may result in an increased reflex include the animal's level of excitement, anxiety, the evaluator's strength and technique, or spinal cord pathology. Furthermore, hyperreflexia does not change the overall lesion localization. Therefore, hyperreflexia will not be discussed in the cases presented in this text. Reduced or absent reflexes will be discussed and indicate a problem in the neuromuscular system. Reflexes performed in the cases discussed in this text are included in Table 2.5.

Cutaneous trunci reflex pathway involves ascending sensory nerves in the skin that are stimulated bilaterally starting at L6 (approximately the cranial aspect of the pelvis). The sensory information ascends bilaterally through the spinal cord, synapses in the C8–T2 spinal cord segment with the lateral thoracic nerve (motor efferent), and the resulting sign is contraction of the cutaneous trunci muscles unilaterally or bilaterally. This pathway is not useful when assessing spinal cord integrity for cats (Paushter *et al.*, 2020).

Table 2.5. Spinal reflexes performed in the neurologic examination in cases included in this text.

	Spinal cord segment	Spinal nerve(s) evaluated
Thoracic limb		
Biceps reflex	C6–C8	Musculocutaneous
Triceps reflex	C7–T1	Radial
Extensor carpi radialis[a]	C7–T1	Radial
Withdrawal	C6–T2	Musculocutaneous and radial
Pelvic limb		
Patellar reflex	L4–L6	Femoral
Gastrocnemius reflex	L7–S1	Tibial branch of sciatic
Cranial tibialis[a]	L6–L7	Peroneal branch of sciatic
Withdrawal	L6–S3	Sciatic
Other		
Perineal	S1–Cd	Pudendal and caudal nerves
Cutaneous trunci[b]	C8–L6[c]	Dorsal sensory nerves and lateral thoracic

[a]Not performed by all neurologists, therefore this reflex may not be discussed in some of the cases in this text.
[b]Not performed on cats.
[c]Dorsal sensory nerves provide innervation from C8 to L6, however this may only extend to L4–L5 in some animals.

Palpation

Palpation is performed with three goals in mind: (i) assess muscle size; (ii) assess muscle pain; and (iii) determine if paraspinal or spinal pain is present. As a rule, one should consider first palpating in areas not suspected to be painful based on the history (e.g., a dog with low head carriage may have neck pain, therefore start with lumbar palpation). When performing palpation, support under the abdomen or inguinal region while providing digital pressure with one finger on each side of the dorsal process in the area of the articular processes. Firm pressure should be applied at each intervertebral disc space moving in a stepwise fashion. If pain is detected, further investigation with additional palpation may be indicated. Identification of painful regions also includes flexion of the neck in all four directions to assess range of motion and pain. Flexion of the neck is not done in patients where you suspect cervical instability or fracture.

Nociception

Deep pain perception is evaluated by applying firm pressure on the toe with a hemostat. Sensory pathways from the point of stimulation to the cerebrum must be intact for a conscious response to the stimuli. *A conscious response is required from the patient.* Let's repeat that last sentence, as it's the most important thing in this paragraph: A conscious response is required to confirm the presence of nociception. A conscious response may include vocalization, turning the head/neck toward the area of testing, pupillary dilation, or trying to move away repeatedly when stimulation is applied. Testing for nociception is performed in plegic animals and animals with suspected sensory neuropathies. Note that evidence of the withdrawal reflex is not indication of intact nociception. Take care to identify a separate conscious response, even when withdrawal is present or brisk!

References

de Lahunta, A. and Glass, E. (2009) *Veterinary Neuroanatomy and Clinical Neurology*, 3rd edn. Saunders Elsevier, St. Louis, Missouri.

Paushter, A.M., Hague, D.W., Foss, K.D. and Sander, W.E. (2020) Assessment of the cutaneous trunci muscle reflex in neurologically abnormal cats. *Journal of Feline Medicine and Surgery* 22(12), 1200–1205. doi: 10.1177/1098612X20917810.

Rylander, H. (2013) The neurologic examination in companion animals. *Today's Veterinary Practice* Jan/Feb, 18–22.

3 Neuroanatomic Lesion Localization

Heidi Barnes Heller*

Barnes Veterinary Specialty Services, Madison, Wisconsin, USA

Unless otherwise noted, all images and videos are owned by the lead author.

After completing the neurologic examination, you will need to localize the lesion in order to produce an appropriate list of differential diagnoses and to develop a relevant diagnostic plan. NALL is performed by analyzing all of the information gained by the neurologic examination in combination with the practitioner's knowledge of neuroanatomy. NALL options are listed in Table 3.1.

Table 3.1. Terminology used to describe the neuroanatomic lesion localization for animals.

Terminology	Anatomic group
Prosencephalon	Intracranial
Midbrain/mesencephalon	Intracranial
Pons/metencephalon	Intracranial
Medulla oblongata/myelencephalon	Intracranial
Cerebellum	Intracranial
Any cranial nerve	Intracranial or peripheral neuropathy
C1–C5 myelopathy	Spinal cord
C6–T2 myelopathy	Spinal cord
C6–T2 radiculopathy/neuropathy	Peripheral neuropathy
T3–L3 myelopathy	Spinal cord
L4–S2 myelopathy	Spinal cord
L4–S3 radiculopathy/neuropathy	Peripheral neuropathy
(Poly) neuropathy	Neuromuscular
Neuromuscular junctionopathy	Neuromuscular
Myopathy	Neuromuscular

*Email: barnes@barnesveterinaryservices.com

© CAB International 2022. *Small Animal Neuroanatomic Lesion Localization Practice Book* (ed. H. Barnes Heller)
DOI: 10.1079/9781789247947.0003

Prosencephalon

The following can be abnormal with a lesion in the prosencephalon: Seizures, change in mentation, behavior change, loss of learned response (e.g., house training), circling towards the lesion, aimless pacing or wandering, head pressing, postural reaction deficits contralateral to the lesion, visual deficits contralateral to the lesion with normal PLR, head or trunk twisted ipsilateral to the lesion, and hemi-inattention or neglect of the contralateral side.

Brainstem

Cranial nerve deficits indicate a lesion in the peripheral nerve, or the brainstem segment associated with the cell bodies of that cranial nerve, for all cranial nerves except CN I and CN II. When presented with a patient with a cranial nerve deficit in CN III–XII the practitioner must determine if the lesion is located in the brainstem (i.e., centrally) or in the peripheral nerve itself (i.e., peripherally). Take the following steps to do so:

1. Identify the abnormal test (e.g., absent palpebral reflex).
2. Determine which cranial nerves can be affected (e.g., facial nerve (CN VII) or trigeminal nerve (CN V)).
3. Evaluate other neurologic tests to determine if the disease process is in the motor or sensory portion of the affected reflex(es) (e.g., evaluate the corneal reflex, which involves CN V and CN VI).
4. Identify the segment of brainstem associated with the nucleus of the cranial nerve that is suspected to be abnormal (e.g., medulla oblongata).
5. Identify if any long tract deficits (postural reaction deficits or UMN dysfunction) or mentation changes (obtunded, stupor, coma) are present (e.g., ipsilateral paw replacement deficit, ipsilateral hemiparesis, or obtunded mentation).
    a. If yes, the lesion is in the brainstem. Development of a differential diagnoses list and recommendations for testing should reflect evaluation of brainstem structures (e.g., MRI).
    b. If no, the lesion is in the peripheral nerve or receptor (if sensory) of the affected nerve. Development of a differential diagnoses list and recommendations for testing should reflect disease identification in the peripheral nerve or receptor.

The Vestibular System

The vestibular system is a unique system that often requires greater focus when learning NALL. The same rules of localization discussed for CN III–XII apply to CN VIII; nevertheless this system can be overwhelming for practitioners, therefore Table 3.2 may help clarify the NALL.

Table 3.2. Neuroanatomic lesion localization for the vestibular system.

Examination finding	Peripheral (CN VIII)	Medulla oblongata	Cerebellum
Head tilt	+ (ipsilateral)	+ (ipsilateral)	+ (ipsilateral or contralateral)
Nystagmus	+	+	+
Ataxia	+	+	+
Postural reaction deficits	–	+ (ipsilateral)	+/– (ipsilateral)
UMN paresis	–	+ (ipsilateral)	–
Decreased mentation	–	+	–
Hypermetria	–	–	+ (ipsilateral)
Intention tremors	–	–	+

(+) = this examination finding can be associated with this NALL; (–) = this finding is not associated with this NALL; (+/–) = conflicting information in the literature or in the author's experience exists for this finding in this NALL; ipsilateral = finding is on the same side as the lesion; contralateral = finding is on the opposite side to the lesion.

The Visual System

Evaluation of the visual system is limited to the use of menace response testing, PLR testing, and visual tracking for the cases in this text. Although other tests are available for visual testing, they are not routinely used and not discussed herein. The menace response is a learned response; therefore animals less than 3 months of age may not have developed a menace response. Table 3.3 provides examples of NALL for some of the most common menace and PLR deficits identified in small animals.

Lesion Localization: Spinal Cord

Extradural spinal cord compression results in proprioceptive abnormalities first, followed next by UMN paresis, and lastly by loss of nociception, in that order. If an animal has marked paresis and yet it has intact postural reactions, it is less likely to be a spinal cord lesion and more likely to be a lesion in the peripheral nerve, neuromuscular junction, or muscle (Rylander, 2013).

At times it may be difficult to localize a patient's signs to a peripheral neuropathy versus C6–T2 or L4–S3 spinal cord lesion because both may result in reduced or absent reflexes. Remember that lesions in the C6–T2 spinal cord segment will result in paresis and proprioceptive deficits in the pelvic limbs in addition to the reflex deficits in the affected thoracic limb(s). Furthermore, lesions affecting the cauda equina (L4–S3) do not have evidence of disease in thoracic limbs. Table 3.4 outlines the neurologic examination abnormalities found with lesion localization in the spinal cord segments and neuromuscular system.

How to localize a spinal cord lesion:

1. No mentation changes, seizures, or cranial nerve deficits can be present for a spinal cord lesion.

Table 3.3. Neuroanatomic lesion localization for common menace response and pupillary light reflex deficits.

A lesion is located in….	Menace (OD)	Menace (OS)	Direct PLR OD	Direct PLR OS	Indirect PLR OD	Indirect PLR OS
Right cerebrum	+	–	+	+	+	+
Left cerebrum	–	+	+	+	+	+
Midbrain (brainstem)[a]	+	+	–	–	–	–
Optic chiasm	–	–	–	–	–	–
Right optic nerve (CN II)	–	+	–	+	+	–
Left optic nerve (CN II)	+	–	+	–	–	+

(+) = the neurologic examination finding is present or normal; (–) = the neurologic examination finding is absent or abnormal; direct = light shone in the eye results in pupillary constriction of the eye under evaluation; indirect = light shone in the other eye results in constriction of the eye under evaluation.
[a]Many patients with midbrain lesions are unconscious; therefore menace cannot be performed. However, if not unconscious, the findings would be as listed.

Table 3.4. Neurologic examination abnormalities noted for spinal cord and neuromuscular localization in dogs and cats.

Spinal cord segment	Reflexes	Gait	Postural reactions
C1–C5	Normal all limbs	Tetraparesis/plegia Ataxia all limbs	Affected all limbs
C6–T2	Reduced/absent thoracic Normal pelvic	Tetraparesis/plegia Ataxia pelvic limbs, variable thoracic limbs	Affected pelvic limbs, variable thoracic limbs
T3–L3	Normal all limbs	Paraparesis/plegia Ataxia pelvic limbs	Affected pelvic limbs only
L4–S2	Normal thoracic Reduced/absent pelvic	Paraparesis/plegia Rarely ataxia of the pelvic limbs	Variable pelvic limbs
Peripheral neuropathy	Reduced to absent in thoracic and pelvic limbs	Paraparesis or tetraparesis but no ataxia	Reduced to normal
Neuromuscular junction	Reduced to absent spinal reflexes in thoracic and pelvic limbs	Usually non-ambulatory paresis or plegia. May involve all four limbs or start ascending from just pelvic limbs	Reduced to absent, depending on severity of disease
Myopathy	Normal	Tetraparesis or paraparesis	Normal

2. Determine if just the pelvic limbs are involved, or if one or both thoracic limbs are involved.
  a. If only the pelvic limbs are affected, the lesion must be caudal to T2 (T3–L3 or L4–S3).
  b. If one or both thoracic limbs are involved, the lesion must be CRANIAL to T2 (e.g., C1–C5 or C6–T2).
  c. If the lesion is caudal to T2, determine if pelvic limb reflexes are normal or abnormal.
    i. If abnormal reflexes are present, the lesion is a L4–S3 myelopathy.
    ii. If normal reflexes are present, the lesion is a T3–L3 myelopathy.
  d. If the lesion is cranial to T2, determine if the thoracic limb reflexes are normal or abnormal.
    i. If reflexes are abnormal, the lesion is a C6–T2 myelopathy.
    ii. If the reflexes are normal, the lesion is a C1–C5 myelopathy.
  e. If reflexes are abnormal in both thoracic and pelvic limbs, the NALL may be neuromuscular and not in the spinal cord.
At the end of the neurological exam, you should be able to answer the questions posed in Table 3.5.

Table 3.5. After finishing the neurologic examination, complete this checklist to localize the lesion.

Does the pet have a neurologic problem? Yes or no
If yes, where is the lesion?
- Intracranial
  - Prosencephalon/forebrain
  - Brainstem
    - Midbrain/mesencephalon
    - Pons/metencephalon
    - Medulla oblongata/myelencephalon
  - Cerebellum
  - Peripheral cranial nerve disease
- Spinal cord
  - C1–C5 myelopathy
  - C6–T2 myelopathy
  - T3–L3 myelopathy
  - L4–S3 myelopathy
- Neuromuscular
  - Peripheral nerves
  - Neuromuscular junction
  - Muscle
  - Multifocal CNS
  - Multifocal CNS and PNS

Reference

Rylander, H. (2013) The neurologic examination in companion animals. *Today's Veterinary Practice* Jan/Feb, 18–22.

4 Intracranial Disease

HEIDI BARNES HELLER[1]*, SIMON PLATT[2]
AND HELENA RYLANDER[3]

[1]*Barnes Veterinary Specialty Services, Madison, Wisconsin, USA;*
[2]*Veterinary Neurology Training LLC, Watkinsville, Georgia, USA;*
[3]*University of Wisconsin–Madison, Madison, Wisconsin, USA*

Unless otherwise noted, all images and videos are owned by the lead author.

Case 1

Patient signalment

An 11-year-old male castrated Chihuahua.

History

Five months' history of a head tilt and ataxia; acute onset, static or slightly progressive.

Physical examination

T: 38.8°C/102°F   P: 150 beats/min   R: panting

- **EENT:** Nuclear sclerosis bilaterally with evidence of iris atrophy bilaterally; patent nares.
- **Lymph nodes:** Submandibular, prescapular, and popliteal lymph nodes palpate soft, round, and symmetrical.

*Email: barnes@barnesveterinaryservices.com

© CAB International 2022. *Small Animal Neuroanatomic Lesion Localization Practice Book*
(ed. H. Barnes Heller)
DOI: 10.1079/9781789247947.0004

- **Oropharyngeal:** Moderate to severe periodontal disease; pink mucous membranes; CRT < 2 s.
- **Integument:** Healthy hair coat and skin, no signs of ectoparasites.
- **Musculoskeletal:** Symmetric musculature, medial patella luxation grade 2/4 bilaterally.
- **Abdominal palpation:** Soft abdomen, no organomegaly or masses noted.
- **Urogenital:** Neutered, no discharge from prepuce, normal.
- **Respiratory:** Clear lung sounds in all fields.
- **Cardiac:** Strong synchronous femoral pulses, no murmurs or arrhythmia.

Neurologic examination

- **Mentation:** BAR.
- **Cranial nerve exam:** Left-sided head tilt, ventral strabismus OD in dorsal recumbency, a few beats of rotary nystagmus in dorsal recumbency, all other cranial nerves within normal limits.
- **Spinal reflexes:** All spinal reflexes normal.
- **Postural reactions:** Paw replacement absent in left thoracic and pelvic limbs, delayed to absent in right pelvic limb, and normal in right thoracic limb.
- **Gait assessment:** Ambulatory with mild vestibular ataxia (listing to the left).
- **Spinal palpation:** No apparent pain.
- **Cervical range of motion:** Full range of motion.
- **Other:** None.

Neuroanatomic lesion localization practice sheet

Use this space below to work through NALL for Case 1. When you have finished, turn to the answer section on the following page to check your answers.

Abnormality	Possible NALL	Possible NALL	Possible NALL	Possible NALL	Possible NALL	Possible NALL

Discussion on neuroanatomic lesion localization

Abnormality	Possible NALL	Possible NALL	Possible NALL	Possible NALL
Left-sided head tilt, inducible rotary nystagmus	Peripheral vestibular: Left CN VIII	Central vestibular: Left medulla oblongata	Cerebellum	
Positional strabismus OD	Right peripheral vestibular: Right CN VIII	Right or left central vestibular: Medulla oblongata	Cerebellum	
Vestibular ataxia, listing to the left	Peripheral vestibular: Left CN VIII	Central vestibular: Left medulla oblongata		
Absent paw replacement left thoracic and pelvic limb, and delayed to absent right pelvic limb	C6–T2 spinal cord segments	C1–C5 spinal cord segments	Left brainstem (medulla, pons, or midbrain)	Right prosencephalon

Neuroanatomic lesion localization, Case 1: Left brainstem vestibular

This patient has vestibular syndrome: vestibular ataxia, head tilt, strabismus, and spontaneous nystagmus. The vestibular signs do not help localizing the lesion to the peripheral or the central vestibular system. Other, nonvestibular findings on our neurologic examination will help us localizing the lesion. The three nonvestibular findings on our neurologic examination that help us localizing the lesion to the brainstem and thus the central vestibular system are mentation change, other cranial nerve deficits, and postural reaction deficits.

Postural reactions involve long pathways: The sensory nerve in the skin, sensory nerve up along the limb, through the ascending spinal cord tracts and through the brainstem, to the contralateral prosencephalon. The motor cortex sends impulses through the descending motor pathways through the brainstem and spinal cord to the peripheral motor nerves. There are many pathways participating in the postural reaction tests, and they decussate at different levels in the spinal cord and brainstem. The summary of all those decussations is that in the majority of cases the postural reactions are affected ipsilateral to a lesion in the brainstem and contralateral to a lesion in the prosencephalon.

The RAS in the brainstem is part of the reticular formation and is crucial for our behavioral arousal, alertness, awareness, and motivation. Therefore, a lesion in the brainstem may cause a mentation change.

The nuclei of CN V–XII are located in the medulla, and can be affected with a lesion in the medulla oblongata with cranial nerve deficits as a result.

Not all dogs with central vestibular syndrome have any of these three abnormalities. However, if one of these is present, the vestibular dysfunction can be localized to the brainstem. The postural reaction deficits are always ipsilateral to the lesion. The paw replacement deficit in the right pelvic limb may be due to a lesion in the T3–L3 spinal cord segment in addition to the central vestibular lesion; or could be from a left-sided brainstem lesion that extends over slightly to the right side, thus affecting the proprioceptive pathways from the right pelvic limb.

Differential diagnoses

Going through the DAMNITV scheme and thinking about possible differential diagnoses, the most likely, given the static or slowly progressive signs, the 5-month history, and the age of the dog, are: Neoplasia (primary or metastatic), inflammatory (MUO), infectious (fungal, protozoal, bacterial, viral).

Diagnostic testing and results

- **CBC:** No significant abnormalities.
- **Chemistry panel:** No significant abnormalities.
- **Total T4:** Within normal range.
- **Thoracic radiographs:** No signs of metastatic disease or infection.
- **MRI (brain):** Intracranial, extra-axial, strongly contrast-enhancing left-sided brainstem mass. Differential diagnoses: Meningioma, histiocytic sarcoma, fungal granuloma (Fig. 4.1).
- **CSF analysis (cisternal):** Total protein = 51.0 mg/dl ($n < 25$), RBCs = 2 cells/µl, TNCC = 4 cells/µl ($n < 5$), lymphocytes = 47 %, eosinophils = 1 %, mononuclear cells = 52 %.

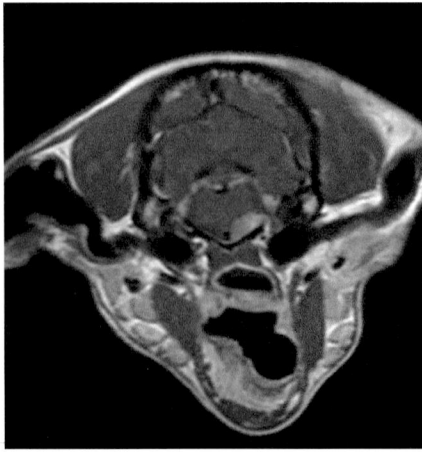

Fig. 4.1. Transverse T1W image post contrast at the level of the ears and pons in Case 1. Contrast-enhancing mass under the left brainstem. This mass extended from the midbrain to the medulla oblongata. (Image used with permission from Dr. Helena Rylander.)

Case conclusion

The CSF analysis showed a mild increase in protein content, but no evidence of inflammation. Given this finding, a fungal granuloma or a bacterial infection was not likely. There was no evidence of lymphoma in the CSF sample. An increase in protein content is common when there is a space-occupying lesion in the brain or the spinal cord. Therefore, this dog was diagnosed with a neoplastic mass affecting the left lateral aspect of the brainstem. Treatment options may include palliative treatment, radiation therapy, or surgical removal. Each of these treatment modalities has a variable survival rate (Rossmeisl et al., 2013; Van Asselt et al., 2020). In this case the clients elected palliative care.

Case 2

Patient signalment

A 10-month-old male castrated Boxer mix.

History

A few weeks' history of increased anxiety/reclusive behavior and worsening of submissive/inappropriate urination with any interaction. Acute onset of mentation change and nonambulation in the past 24 h, with progressive worsening.

Physical examination

T: 38.1°C /100.7°F   P: 112 beats/min   R: 80 breaths/min

- **EENT:** No oculonasal discharge or aural debris.
- **Lymph nodes:** Mandibular, prescapular, and popliteal lymph nodes smooth and symmetric.
- **Oropharyngeal:** Clean teeth and normal gingiva, pink mucous membranes, CRT = 2 s.
- **Integument:** Clean shiny hair coat; no alopecia, redness, or signs of ectoparasites.
- **Musculoskeletal:** No joint swelling or long bone pain.
- **Abdominal palpation:** Soft, nonpainful, no masses or organomegaly noted.
- **Urogenital:** Normal external genitalia, castrated male.
- **Respiratory:** Intermittent tachypnea, normal bronchovesicular sounds in all lung fields.
- **Cardiac:** Intermittent tachycardia/bradycardia, strong synchronous femoral pulses, no murmurs or arrhythmia.

Neurologic examination

- **Mentation:** Obtunded, progressed during examination from moderate obtundation to intermittently stuporous.
- **Cranial nerve exam:** Spontaneous vertical nystagmus, unchanging with head positioning, anisocoria with miosis OD, absent gag reflex.
- **Spinal reflexes:** All within normal limits.
- **Postural reactions:** Absent paw replacement all limbs.
- **Gait assessment:** Nonambulatory tetraparesis; in lateral recumbency, persistent cervical extension, intermittent opisthotonos with extensor rigidity in all limbs (thoracic limbs worse than pelvic limbs).
- **Spinal palpation:** No apparent pain.
- **Cervical range of motion:** Vocalizes and flinches on attempt to perform ventral cervical flexion.
- **Other:** None.

Neuroanatomic lesion localization practice sheet

Use this space below to work through NALL for Case 2. When you have finished, turn to the answer section on the following page to check your answers.

Abnormality	Possible NALL	Possible NALL	Possible NALL	Possible NALL	Possible NALL	Possible NALL

Discussion on neuroanatomic lesion localization

Abnormality	Possible NALL	Possible NALL	Possible NALL	Possible NALL	Possible NALL	Possible NALL
Obtunded	Prosencephalon	Midbrain	Pons	Medulla oblongata		
Opisthotonos		Midbrain		Cerebellum		
Vertical nystagmus			Inner ear peripheral CN VIII (left or right side)	Medulla oblongata (left or right side)		
Anisocoria with miosis OD and intact PLR			Loss of sympathetic innervation (Horner's syndrome)			
Absent gag reflex	Peripheral CN IX and CN X			Medulla oblongata		
Nonambulatory tetraparesis	Prosencephalon	Brainstem	C1–C5 spinal cord segments	C6–T2 spinal cord segments	Peripheral nerve	Neuromuscular junction
Absent paw replacement all limbs	Prosencephalon	Brainstem	C1–C5 spinal cord segments	C6–T2 spinal cord segments	Peripheral nerve	Neuromuscular junction

Neuroanatomic lesion localization, Case 2: Brainstem with possible cerebellar herniation

Mentation change (obtunded, stupor, coma) indicates a lesion in the prosencephalon or brainstem. The RAS in the brainstem is responsible for our awareness and level of alertness.

The opisthotonos described in this case is suggestive of cerebellar lesion localization due to the increased muscle tone of all four limbs. Opisthotonos can also be noted with midbrain lesions; however with midbrain lesion localization, muscle tone is typically increased in the thoracic limbs only.

The spontaneous vertical nystagmus indicates a lesion in the vestibular system. Although the direction of the nystagmus does not define if the lesion is in the peripheral or central vestibular system, vertical nystagmus is more common in central vestibular syndrome than in peripheral vestibular syndrome.

Anisocoria means pupils of different sizes. In this case it was concluded that the right eye was miotic. If you examine the eyes in the dark and the pupil does not dilate, the miotic pupil is the abnormal one. If one pupil appears larger than expected in daylight, that pupil would be mydriatic and the abnormal pupil.

Miosis in patients with severe brain lesions is a sign of increased intracranial pressure and needs to be taken seriously.

CN IX (glossopharyngeal nerve) and CN X (vagus nerve) innervate the larynx, where CN X is the sensory (afferent) nerve and CN IX the motor (efferent) nerve. The nuclei of these nerves are located in the medulla oblongata.

Postural reactions involve long pathways: The sensory nerve in the skin, sensory nerve up along the limb, through the ascending spinal cord tracts and through the brainstem, to the contralateral prosencephalon. The motor cortex sends impulses through the descending motor pathways through the brainstem and spinal cord to the peripheral motor nerves. There are many pathways participating in the postural reaction tests, and they decussate at different levels in the spinal cord and brainstem. The summary of all those decussations is that in the majority of cases the postural reactions are affected ipsilateral to a lesion in the brainstem and contralateral to a lesion in the prosencephalon. Absent postural reactions in all limbs can be caused by a lesion anywhere cranial to the thoracic limbs, i.e., the cervical spinal cord or the brain.

Differential diagnoses

- **Anomalous:** A vascular malformation causing compression, or a secondary hemorrhagic infarct; hydrocephalus; supracollicular fluid accumulation (quadrigeminal cyst); epidermoid cyst.
- **Neoplasia:** Nephroblastoma—this is a primitive neuroectodermal tumor originating from fetal neurons that are left behind in the mature brain.
- **Infection:** Fungal, protozoal, less likely bacterial or viral (bacterial is less common and viral usually does not result in a space-occupying lesion).
- **Inflammatory:** Such as MUO.
- **Vascular:** Hemorrhagic or ischemic infarct (spontaneous or secondary to a vascular malformation or an infection).

Diagnostic testing and results

The patient was treated with mannitol at 1 g/kg IV as a bolus to reduce the brain edema and reduce the intracranial pressure. A temporary improvement in mentation was noted.

The patient was anesthetized for an MRI of the brain (Fig. 4.2). The MRI showed an obstructive hydrocephalus due to a malformation of the mesencephalic aqueduct (obstruction of the aqueduct), periventricular edema, and secondary cerebellar herniation. The periventricular edema was most likely due to a rapid increase in intracranial pressure.

Case conclusion

Congenital hydrocephalus is most often due to a malformation and obstruction of the mesencephalic aqueduct in the mesencephalon (midbrain). Neurologic

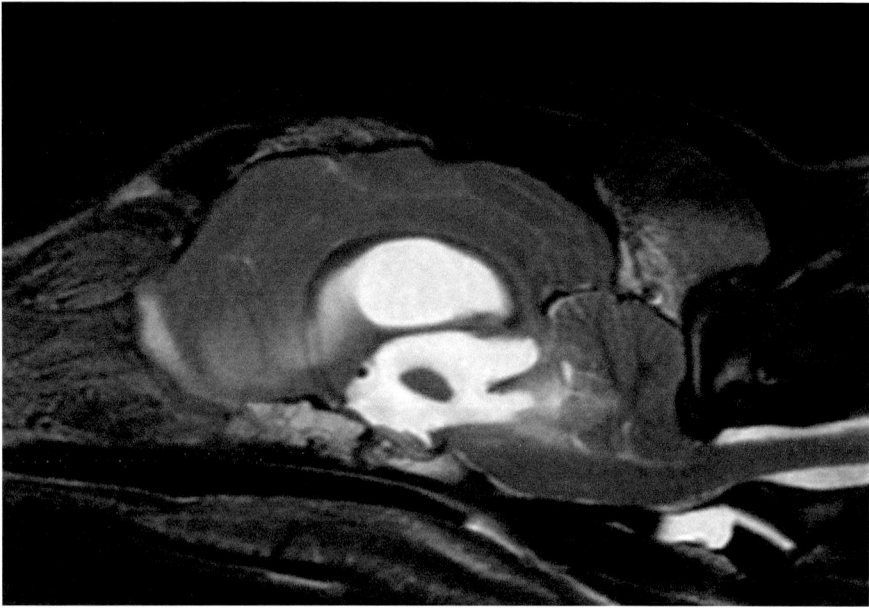

Fig. 4.2. Sagittal T2W image of the brain in Case 2. There is enlargement of the lateral ventricles and third ventricle, periaqueductal edema, and cerebellar herniation. (Image used with permission from Dr. Helena Rylander.)

signs from compression of the prosencephalon are obtundation, circling and postural reaction deficits, and sometimes seizures. In some cases, the neurologic signs become obvious only when the hydrocephalus results in compression of the brainstem and cerebellar herniation.

In this case, an acute surgery was necessary with placement of a ventriculoperitoneal shunt, which drains CSF from the ventricular system to the abdomen (Gradner *et al.*, 2019; Schmidt *et al.*, 2019). This owner declined any treatment and elected humane euthanasia.

Case 3

Patient signalment

An 11-year-old male castrated domestic short-haired cat.

History

Four-month history of slowly progressive signs including decreased interaction with owners and decreased jumping up on chairs. A sudden onset of more obvious mentation change was noted a few days prior to examination.

Physical examination

T: 38.7°C/101.8°F   P: 180 beats/min   R: 24 breaths/min

- **BCS:** 3/9.
- **EENT:** Clean ear, clear cornea, no aural or ocular discharge.
- **Lymph nodes:** Submandibular, prescapular, and popliteal lymph nodes all soft, symmetric and of normal size.
- **Oropharyngeal:** Moderate dental tartar, gingiva pink, no masses noted.
- **Integument:** Full hair coat; no hair loss, redness, seborrhea, or ectoparasites noted.
- **Musculoskeletal:** Lean body condition, symmetric musculature.
- **Abdominal palpation:** Soft, nonpainful, no organomegaly or masses noted.
- **Urogenital:** Castrated male, normal.
- **Respiratory:** Eupneic, no crackles or wheezes.
- **Cardiac:** Strong synchronous femoral pulses, no arrhythmia. Grade III/VI left systolic murmur.

Neurologic examination

- **Mentation:** Moderate obtundation, randomly sniffs the floor.
- **Cranial nerve exam:** No abnormalities detected.
- **Spinal reflexes:** All within normal limits.
- **Postural reactions:** Paw replacement absent right thoracic and right pelvic limbs, normal left side.
- **Gait assessment:** Ambulatory tetraparesis; circles to the left, stops suddenly, and stands with body turned to the left (Video 4.1).
- **Spinal palpation:** No apparent pain.
- **Cervical range of motion:** Full range of motion of the neck.
- **Other:** Does not react to painful stimulus on the right side of the body, is able to localize pain stimulus on the left side of the body. This is called right hemineglect.

Video 4.1. Eleven-year-old male castrated domestic short-haired cat, Case 3. Gait assessment video showing circling left, with ambulatory tetraparesis and body turn left. (Video used with permission from Dr. Helena Rylander.) (https://vimeo.com/696921790; video.cabi.org/VBSVT)

Neuroanatomic lesion localization practice sheet

Use this space below to work through NALL for Case 3. When you have finished, turn to the answer section on the following page to check your answers.

Abnormality	Possible NALL	Possible NALL	Possible NALL	Possible NALL	Possible NALL	Possible NALL

Discussion on neuroanatomic lesion localization

Abnormality	Possible NALL	Possible NALL	Possible NALL	Possible NALL
Obtunded	Prosencephalon	Midbrain	Pons	Medulla
Circles to the left, without a head tilt	Left prosencephalon			
Body turn to the left	Left prosencephalon			
Paw replacement absent right side	Left prosencephalon	Midbrain	Right pons	Right medulla
Right-sided hemineglect	Left prosencephalon			

Neuroanatomic lesion localization, Case 3: Left prosencephalon

Mentation change (obtunded, stupor, coma) indicates a lesion in the prosencephalon or brainstem. The RAS in the brainstem is responsible for our awareness and level of alertness.

Animals circle toward the side of the lesion, regardless of if the lesion is in the prosencephalon or the brainstem. Circling due to brainstem localization is due to dysfunction affecting the vestibular system. A head tilt is expected concurrently with circling due to brainstem localization. Circling in the case of a lesion in the prosencephalon is most likely due to hemineglect—the patient circles toward the side of the world that it recognizes. Hemineglect can be identified if the patient is aware of only one side of the world and thus turns in that direction. Hemineglect is always due to a lesion in the prosencephalon. When you pinch one side of the body to elicit pain, the patient may feel it but not be able to localize the origin of the pain stimulus. The left prosencephalon controls recognition of the right side of the body and face. With a lesion in the left prosencephalon, the patient may not be aware or recognize the right side of the world.

Postural reactions involve long pathways: The sensory nerve in the skin, sensory nerve up along the limb, through the ascending spinal cord tracts and through the brainstem, to the contralateral prosencephalon. The motor cortex sends impulses through the descending motor pathways through the brainstem and spinal cord to the peripheral motor nerves. There are many pathways participating in the postural reaction tests, and they decussate at different levels in the spinal cord and brainstem. The summary of all those decussations is that in the majority of cases the postural reactions are affected ipsilateral to a lesion in the brainstem and contralateral to a lesion in the prosencephalon.

Differential diagnoses

Neoplasia, infection, inflammation.

Neoplasia, either primary or metastatic, is the most likely differential diagnosis given the slowly progressive history and the age of the cat. The most common brain tumors in cats are meningioma and lymphoma and are considered most likely for this case. Metastatic neoplasia is less common but can arise from any thoracic or abdominal mass.

Infection is more common than inflammatory/immune-mediated diseases in cats, however both should be included as differential diagnoses for this cat. Toxoplasma, FIP, *Cryptococcus* and blastomycosis could be considered likely infectious diseases resulting in clinical signs and progression. Infectious meningoencephalitis rarely builds in severity slowly over 5 months, therefore this was considered less likely for this cat.

Diagnostic testing and results

A CBC showed a mild nonregenerative anemia of chronic disease. A chemistry panel did not reveal significant abnormalities. Thoracic radiographs and abdominal ultrasound were normal for the age of the cat. An ECG showed changes consistent with mild hypertrophic cardiomyopathy.

An MRI of the brain showed a large mass in the left prosencephalon (Fig. 4.3). The mass had characteristics typical of a meningioma. The mass was causing compression of the left prosencephalon (which was almost absent), a mass effect with shift of the midline, and compression of the right prosencephalon and both lateral ventricles. There was also compression of the left midbrain.

Case conclusion

In this case, the owners elected surgery. The mass was successfully removed. Three days postoperatively the cat was bright and alert and was exploring the exam room. He was discharged to the owner 4 days postoperatively. At home, the cat started jumping up on chairs and interacting with the owners. The

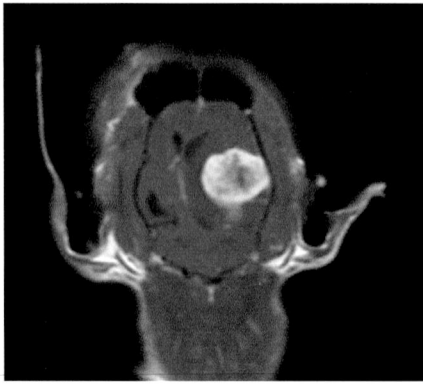

Fig. 4.3. T1W image post IV contrast, dorsal view, in Case 3. There is a strongly homogeneously contrast-enhancing mass on the left side causing mass effect, right shift of the falx cerebri, and compression of the lateral ventricles. Note the hyperostosis adjacent to the mass. (Image used with permission from Dr. Helena Rylander.)

owners reported that the cat was doing well with no recurrence of signs 2 years postoperatively.

Meningiomas in cats are slow growing and respond poorly to radiation therapy. Because of the slow growth, the brain adapts and compensates for a long time, and the mass is usually very large once the neurologic signs become more obvious (Cameron *et al.*, 2015; Korner *et al.*, 2019).

Case 4

Patient signalment

A 7-year-old female spayed Boxer.

History

The dog presented with a 2-week history of lethargy, inappetence, and a fever. In the past week, she had developed a head tilt. Over the last 2 days the owner noticed that the dog had started to stumble occasionally. There had been no change in the dog's behavior or thirst. The dog had been systemically healthy up until this time apart from a grade II/VI heart murmur diagnosed at 4 years of age. The dog was routinely vaccinated and up to date on its parasite prophylaxis. There was no known access to toxins and there was no known traumatic event preceding the clinical signs. The owners reported a recent travel history to the North Carolina mountains, where the dog went on daily hikes.

Physical examination

T: 39.8°C/103.7°F   P: 120 beats/min   R: panting

- **EENT:** No abnormalities noted.
- **Lymph nodes:** No lymphadenopathy noted.
- **Oropharyngeal:** No significant abnormalities.
- **Integument:** One tick between the third and fourth digits of the right thoracic limb, which was then manually removed. No other clinically significant abnormalities noted.
- **Musculoskeletal:** No joint swelling or long bone pain.
- **Abdominal palpation:** No abnormalities noted.
- **Urogenital:** Normal.
- **Respiratory:** No abnormalities detected.
- **Cardiac:** Grade II left systolic heart murmur with normal synchronous pulses. No other abnormalities detected.

Neurologic examination

- **Mentation:** Alert, appropriate to routine stimuli.
- **Cranial nerve exam:** Left head tilt, positional vertical nystagmus, and ventral strabismus OS, all remaining cranial nerves were normal.
- **Spinal reflexes:** All within normal limits.
- **Postural reactions:** Absent proprioceptive deficits in the left thoracic and left pelvic limbs.
- **Gait assessment:** Ambulatory without evidence of paresis, ataxia, or lameness.
- **Spinal palpation:** No apparent pain on palpation.
- **Cervical range of motion:** No abnormalities noted.
- **Other:** None.

Neuroanatomic lesion localization practice sheet

Use this space below to work through NALL for Case 4. When you have finished, turn to the answer section on the following page to check your answers.

Abnormality	Possible NALL	Possible NALL	Possible NALL	Possible NALL	Possible NALL	Possible NALL

Discussion on neuroanatomic lesion localization

Abnormality	Possible NALL	Possible NALL	Possible NALL	Possible NALL	Possible NALL	Possible NALL	Possible NALL	Possible NALL
Left head tilt	Peripheral CN VIII (left)	Medulla (left)	Cerebellum					
Vertical nystagmus	Peripheral CN VIII	Medulla	Cerebellum					
Positional strabismus OS	Peripheral CN VIII (left)	Medulla (left)	Cerebellum					
Absent paw replacement	Prosencephalon (right)	Midbrain (left or right)	Pons (left)	Medulla (left)	C1–C5 spinal cord segments (left)	C6–T2 spinal cord segments (left)	Peripheral nerve	Neuromuscular junction

Neuroanatomic lesion localization, Case 4: Left medulla oblongata

The head tilt is suggestive of a lesion affecting the vestibular system. The vestibular system comprises the peripheral nerve (CN VIII), the brainstem (nucleus located in the medulla), and the cerebellar coordination centers. Vertical nystagmus is suggestive of central localization but should not be used as a sole localizing feature. Postural deficits, mentation changes, and evidence of ipsilateral paresis are key features used to identify peripheral versus central lesions when cranial nerve deficits are identified. The presence of postural deficits in the left pelvic and thoracic limbs in this dog is indicative of brainstem disease affecting the left side, which is further supported by the left-sided head tilt. The presence of positional ventral strabismus in the left eye is also indicative of a left-sided vestibular disease. Overall, a left-sided central vestibular lesion localization was made based on the examination. The normal mentation suggests that the lesion is not damaging the ascending RAS which is so often seen with brainstem diseases (Bongartz et al., 2020).

Differential diagnoses

The clinical signs are chronic and progressive, making a vascular event unlikely. There is no history or evidence of trauma, nutritional deficits, or toxin, making these disease processes also highly unlikely. Metabolic disease is rarely asymmetrical, and the presence of systemic signs (pyrexia) rules out degenerative or anomalous disease. Therefore, the most reasonable differential diagnoses for this case are inflammatory brain disease or neoplasia.

Diagnostic testing and results

CBC, chemistry profile, and urinalysis are highly indicated in this case given the systemic signs. A thorough ophthalmologic examination should be performed in every neurologic case to look for evidence of fundic changes or uveitis compatible with inflammatory disease. Diagnostic testing in an animal determined to have central vestibular disease should include advanced imaging of the brain, preferably MRI, to identify any structural abnormalities. Analysis of CSF collected from the cerebellomedullary cistern can be helpful. However, if any abnormality is identified on imaging that suggests an increased intracranial pressure, such as a mass effect (shifting of structures across the midline), CSF may not be collected because of the risk of fatal brain herniation. When collected, CSF is tested for evidence of inflammation and increased protein concentration. Serological ± CSF testing for potential infectious agents is indicated where CSF testing shows inflammation.

- **CBC:** anemia, mild thrombocytopenia, and leukocytosis characterized by a mature neutrophilia (with toxic change) and leukocytosis.

- **Serum biochemistry profile:** Hypoalbuminemia.
- **MRI:** Normal.
- **CSF analysis:** Mild mononuclear inflammation was seen in CSF with a WBC count calculated to be 27 cells/µl (normal, < 5 cells/µl) and a protein level of 32 mg/dl (normal, < 20 mg/dl).
- **Ophthalmic exam:** Indicated retinal hemorrhages and episcleral injection bilaterally.
- **Immunofluorescent antibody titer for tick-borne disease:** 1:1024 IgG titer for Rocky Mountain spotted fever was noted.
- **Coagulation assays:** Including a buccal mucosal bleeding time, were normal.

Case conclusion

The dog was treated with doxycycline at 10 mg/kg for 2 weeks and an anti-inflammatory prednisone tapering therapy over the same time. Steroid therapy is a controversial therapy in infectious cases; however, given the thrombocytopenia, ocular changes, and neurologic involvement, prednisone was recommended for presumed vasculitis. The dog recovered fully, although her head tilt did not resolve until 8 weeks after therapy.

Rickettsia rickettsii is the causative agent of Rocky Mountain spotted fever. The disease has been documented in dogs and humans throughout the USA, although the incidence is higher in the eastern half of the country, with the southeast having the highest incidence. *R. rickettsii* is transmitted by *Dermacentor* ticks. *Dermacentor andersoni* is the primary vector in the western USA and Canada, whereas *Dermacentor variabilis* is the primary vector in the Midwest and eastern portions of the USA although it is also present in the western USA.

Transmission of *R. rickettsii* from tick to host usually does not occur for a minimum of 5–20 h after attachment, thus prompt removal of attached ticks may prevent infection. *R. rickettsii* invades small blood vessels and replicates in endothelial cells. Damage to endothelial cells results in vasculitis and activation of platelets and the coagulation system. Necrotizing vasculitis may occur through complement activation, cellular chemotaxis, and subsequent extravasation of blood. Severe neurologic dysfunction is associated with the highest IgG titers (>1:1024), and these include rapidly progressing meningoencephalitis causing vestibular dysfunction, seizures, and hyperesthesia (Mikszewski and Vite, 2005).

Case 5

Patient signalment

A 9-month-old male Bengal cat.

History

The cat presented following an approximately 6-month history of ataxia. Onset of the incoordination had been seen when the cat was about 6 weeks of age and since this age there had been no notable progression of the condition. There was only one littermate known (also male) who was normal. There had been no apparent problem with the birth and no access to any toxins or noted trauma during the first weeks of life. The incoordination was manifested by a wide-based stance in the pelvic limbs, hypermetria of all four limbs, and frequent falling with no loss of strength. The owner had also noted an exaggerated head movement when the cat was eating. Although the cat's appetite and thirst were considered normal, the manner in which the cat prehended its food was not and was notably 'messier' in eating than its brother. The cat was considered otherwise to be systemically well and had been routinely vaccinated at 12 weeks of age.

Physical examination

- **EENT:** No oculonasal discharge or aural debris.
- **Lymph nodes:** No abnormalities detected.
- **Oropharyngeal:** No clinically significant abnormalities.
- **Integument:** No clinically significant abnormalities.
- **Musculoskeletal:** Full orthopedic exam not performed. No abnormalities detected.
- **Abdominal palpation:** No abnormalities detected.
- **Urogenital:** Normal.
- **Respiratory:** No clinically significant abnormalities.
- **Cardiac:** No abnormalities detected.

Neurologic examination

- **Mentation:** Alert, responsive.
- **Cranial nerve exam:** Positional, variably rotational nystagmus, absent menace response OU without evidence of blindness, remaining cranial nerve examination was normal.
- **Spinal reflexes:** All within normal ranges.
- **Postural reactions:** Normal hopping in all limbs and normal extensor postural thrust.
- **Gait assessment:** The cat's ability to ambulate was observed revealing a tendency to fall to either side, no loss of strength or dragging of the limbs, and a generalized course tremor, particularly noted when the cat tried to eat; this was considered to be an intention tremor. There was also hypermetria of all four limbs (Video 4.2).
- **Spinal palpation:** No apparent pain.
- **Cervical range of motion:** Not evaluated.
- **Other:** None.

Video 4.2. Nine-month-old Bengal cat in Case 5 demonstrating a generalized course tremor consistent with an intention tremor. (Video used with permission from Dr. Simon Platt.) (https://vimeo.com/696921815; video.cabi.org/WXWHW)

Neuroanatomic lesion localization practice sheet

Use this space below to work through NALL for Case 5. When you have finished, turn to the answer section on the following page to check your answers.

Abnormality	Possible NALL	Possible NALL	Possible NALL	Possible NALL	Possible NALL	Possible NALL

Discussion on neuroanatomic lesion localization

Abnormality	Possible NALL	Possible NALL	Possible NALL	Possible NALL	Possible NALL
Vertical nystagmus	Peripheral CN VIII	Brainstem (medulla)	Cerebellum		
Absent menace	Bilateral CN II	Optic chiasm	Forebrain/ prosencephalon	Facial nerve (CN VII) bilateral	Ocular disease
Hypermetria	Cerebellum	Ascending spinal cord tracts			
Intention tremor	Cerebellum				

Neuroanatomic lesion localization, Case 5: Cerebellum, including the cerebellovestibular nuclei

Evidence of vestibular disease was identified in the form of nystagmus in this cat. Vestibular disease may be a result of damage to the peripheral vestibular system (CN VIII), brainstem (medulla), or cerebellum. The next question is how to localize the lesion within the vestibular system? Paw replacement deficits, hemiparesis, and/or abnormal mentation are common with a brainstem lesion localization, and this cat did not have any of those findings. Furthermore, the intention tremor and hypermetric gait abnormality are only noted with cerebellar damage or disease. To explain all the clinical signs, a lesion of the cerebellum must be considered. The cerebellum has an important function in controlling and moderating movements of the limbs, body, and head, and in the unconscious maintenance of balance. Diffuse cerebellar lesions will therefore result in a loss of this moderating influence and interfere with the unconscious maintenance of balance, with clinical signs of:

- Symmetrical ataxia with no loss of strength.
- Dysmetric gait (altered rate, range, or force of movement), usually with an exaggerated limb movement (hypermetria) but in some instances decreased limb movements (hypometria).
- Truncal ataxia and even a truncal sway.
- Head tremor.
- Muscle hypertonia.
- Vestibular signs will be seen.
- Bilateral menace response deficits in the presence of intact vision and facial nerve function.

Ataxia or incoordination can be due to a vestibular system, sensory system, or cerebellar abnormality. A sensory system abnormality implies a problem of the sensory pathways in the spinal cord or sensory nerves. The latter is extremely rare and is not accompanied by exaggerated movements of the head. Spinal cord abnormalities should be accompanied by postural deficits which were not present in this cat. Most cats with spinal cord diseases are also weak, which again was not evident in this cat.

The menace deficit was attributed to the cerebellar lesion localization in this cat; however, it should be noted that juvenile cats and dogs may not have a normal menace response up to 16 weeks of age. This is a learned response, not a reflex, therefore the cat or dog must develop the awareness in order to respond appropriately to this test.

Differential diagnoses

The age at onset and NALL are highly suggestive of cerebellar hypoplasia; however, an abiotrophy, inflammatory, or infectious meningoencephalitis cannot be fully excluded (Penderis, 2009).

Diagnostic testing and results

The identification of a cerebellar abnormality will usually imply the presence of an intracranial cerebellar lesion. Unlike forebrain disease the cerebellum is not usually affected by metabolic causes, however a number of systemic diseases (including infectious causes) may demonstrate cerebellar signs as the primary presenting clinical sign. Despite the unlikely potential for a metabolic cause, routine bloodwork and a urinalysis are still included in the investigation and were considered normal in this case. This is primarily performed in order to identify any systemic cause, but also to ensure that there is no metabolic contraindication if a general anesthetic is planned.

CSF analysis will help to rule out inflammatory diseases of the nervous system; this was completely normal in this case. MRI (Fig. 4.4) can demonstrate structural abnormalities of the CNS and in this case, they revealed the only abnormality to be a smaller cerebellum with a more prominent overlying CSF signal when compared to a normal age-matched cat. The MRI results, along with the results of the CSF tap, are findings compatible with a condition called cerebellar hypoplasia (Hecht and Adams, 2010).

Case conclusion

There was no progression upon reexamination at 1 and 2 months later, which is an extremely cost-effective method of determining the presence of hypoplasia as the other conditions (such as abiotrophy and inflammatory brain disease) would be expected to display progression (Lowrie, 2021).

In utero or perinatal infection of kittens with feline panleukopenia virus results in marked destruction of the developing cerebellum, particularly the

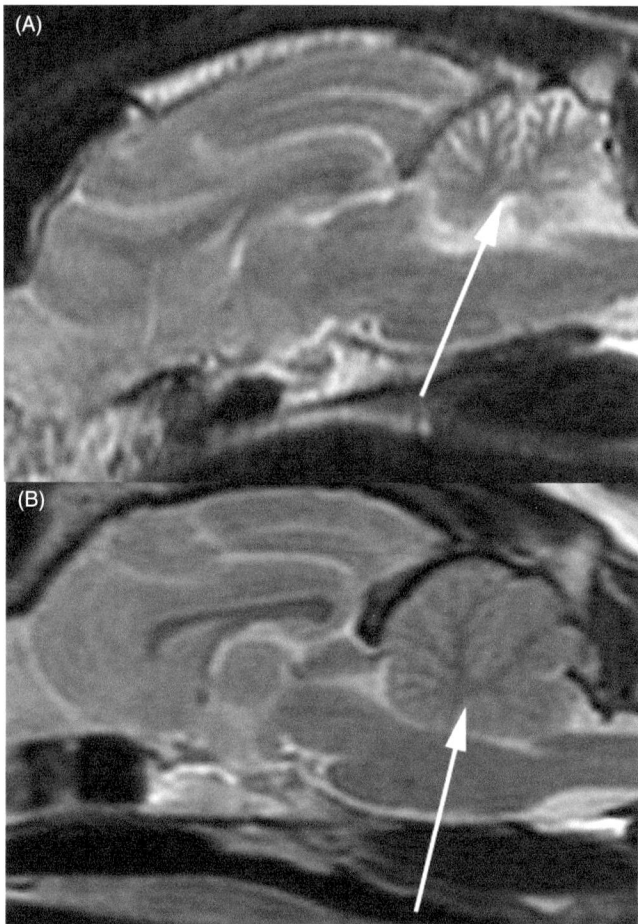

Fig. 4.4. (A) A T2W sagittal image of the brain of the cat in Case 5 compared to an age-matched normal cat (B). Notice the marked prominence of the cerebellar folia due to increased CSF signal compatible with a hypoplastic cerebellum in (A) compared to (B). (Images used with permission from Dr. Simon Platt.)

external germinal layer (Poncelet *et al.*, 2013). The disease is characterized by the presence of symmetrical, nonprogressive cerebellar signs that first become apparent at the time of onset of ambulation, in the region of 3 to 4 weeks of age. Infected animals are variably affected (with the severity decreasing with increasing maturity of the cerebellum at the time of infection) and display inco-ordination, spasticity, truncal sway, and usually a fine head tremor. As the animal grows some compensation may take place (using other sensory modalities like vision to compensate for the impaired balance) resulting in a decrease in the severity of the clinical signs, however the clinical signs will persist for the duration of the animal's life (Lamm and Rezabeck, 2008; Stuetzer and Hartmann, 2014). Due to the lack of progression in the cat in this case, this is the most likely diagnosis.

Case 6

Patient signalment

A 4-year-old male neutered Labrador Retriever.

History

The dog was presented with a 1-week history of progressive behavior change and circling to the right. The behavior changes described by the owners included a quieter demeanor, disinterest in what the owners considered the dog's routine, and a recent inability to catch thrown objects or hear sounds when presented on the left side. The dog had been systemically healthy up until this time in its life. The dog was routinely vaccinated and up to date on its parasite prophylaxis. There was no access to toxins that the owners were aware of and there was no known traumatic event preceding the clinical signs.

Physical examination

- **EENT:** No concerning abnormalities.
- **Lymph nodes:** No peripheral lymphadenopathy.
- **Oropharyngeal:** Normal.
- **Integument:** No concerning abnormalities.
- **Musculoskeletal:** No clinical abnormalities.
- **Abdominal palpation:** Soft, nonpainful palpation.
- **Urogenital:** Normal.
- **Respiratory:** No abnormalities detected.
- **Cardiac:** No abnormalities detected.

Neurologic examination

- **Mentation:** Dull and intermittently confused.
- **Cranial nerve exam:** Normal.
- **Spinal reflexes:** Normal tone and reflexes.
- **Postural reactions:** Proprioceptive placing and hopping were reduced on the left thoracic and left pelvic limbs.
- **Gait assessment:** Ambulatory with frequent circling to the right. No ataxia or paresis was noted.
- **Spinal palpation:** No pain on palpation of the neck and thoracolumbar spinal column.
- **Cervical range of motion:** Not performed.
- **Other:** Neck and body were curved to the right.

Neuroanatomic lesion localization practice sheet

Use this space below to work through NALL for Case 6. When you have finished, turn to the answer section on the following page to check your answers.

Abnormality	Possible NALL	Possible NALL	Possible NALL	Possible NALL	Possible NALL	Possible NALL	Possible NALL

Discussion on neuroanatomic lesion localization

Abnormality	Possible NALL	Possible NALL	Possible NALL	Possible NALL	Possible NALL	Possible NALL
Abnormal mentation	Forebrain/ prosencephalon	Brainstem				
Circling right	Forebrain/ prosencephalon					
Reduced left postural reactions	Forebrain/ prosencephalon	Brainstem	C1–C5 myelopathy	C6–T2 myelopathy	Peripheral neuropathy	Neuromuscular junction

Neuroanatomic lesion localization, Case 6: Right forebrain/prosencephalon

The neurologic examination was suggestive of a lesion affecting the right forebrain. Abnormal mentation (disinterest in activities, confusion, inability to perceive visual/auditory stimuli, and a reduced level of consciousness such as dullness) is indicative of a lesion cranial to the midbrain. The lesion was further lateralized to the right based on the curvature to the right, circling to the right, and the left-sided proprioceptive deficits. Left-sided proprioceptive deficits in both the thoracic and pelvic limbs can indicate a lesion in the left cervical spinal cord, the left brainstem, or the right forebrain. Without obvious motor deficits or cranial nerve deficits, they are more indicative of a forebrain lesion. Motor deficits are not usually seen with forebrain disease, nor does it typically cause pronounced ataxia.

Differential diagnoses

The differential diagnoses for a lesion causing a chronic progressive lateralizing forebrain lesion include inflammatory (infectious or sterile/immune dysfunction) disease and neoplasia. Neoplasia can be primarily affecting the brain (commonly a meningioma or glioma), or secondarily affecting the brain as a metastasis or a tumor of the skull, nose, or ear cavity.

Diagnostic testing and results

- **Minimum database (hematology, serum chemistry, urinalysis):** Normal.
- **Thoracic and abdominal radiographs:** Normal.
- **Abdominal ultrasonography:** Normal.
- **MRI (brain):** Multifocal forebrain disease, predominantly affecting the right cerebrum (Fig. 4.5).
- **CSF analysis (atlanto-occipital cistern):** Protein = 29 mg/dl (normal, < 20 mg/dl), WBCs = 256 cells/µl (normal, < 5 cells/µl), and no RBCs.
- **Infectious disease serum titers:** Performed for *Toxoplasma*, *Neospora*, canine distemper virus, and *Cryptococcus*, all negative.
- **Meningoencephalitis** was diagnosed based on the abnormal MRI and CSF results. All titers were negative and, as such, the inflammatory disease was presumed to be sterile (e.g., MUO).

Case conclusion

The dog was started on an immunosuppressive regimen of oral steroids (prednisone 2 mg/kg/day), which he responded to well and so the dose was tapered over the next 4 months. The dog became refractory to the corticosteroids and was adjunctly treated with another immunomodulator (cytosine arabinoside)

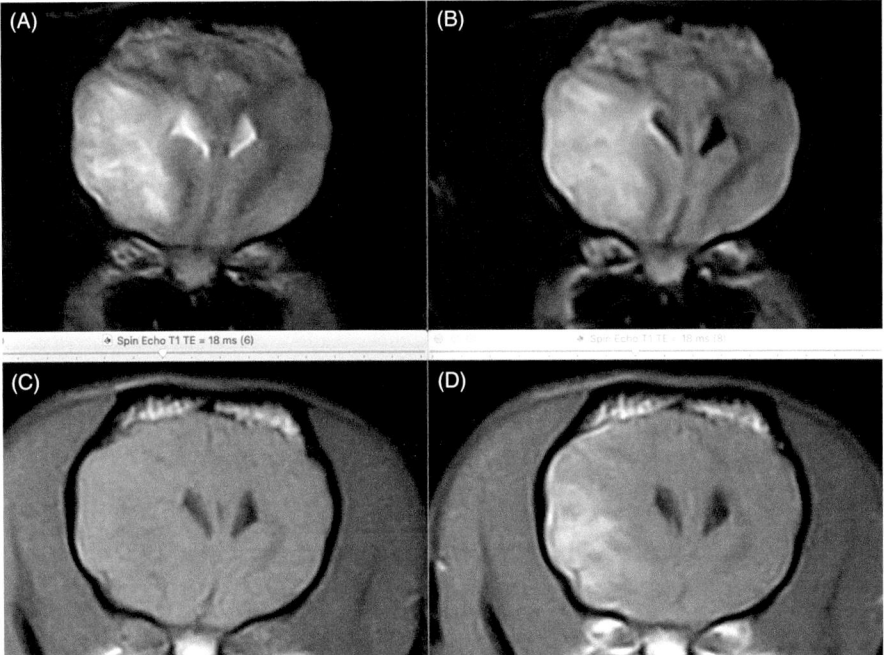

Fig. 4.5. Right cerebrum in Case 6 is hyperintense on the T2W image (A), hyperintense on FLAIR (B), iso- to slightly hypointense on the T1W image pre contrast (C), and patchy contrast enhancement of the region on the T1W post-contrast image is noted (D). (Images used with permission from Dr. Simon Platt.)

parenterally every 3 weeks but began exhibiting seizures, at which time the owner opted to have the dog euthanized. Postmortem confirmed the lesion to be GME.

MUO in the dog comprises a variety of conditions that are thought to be immune mediated in nature and which involve inflammation of the brain, meninges, and/or spinal cord. MUO is the umbrella term used to encompass GME, NLE, and NME (Coates and Jeffery, 2014; Cornelis et al., 2019).

GME is the most common noninfectious inflammatory CNS disease. The clinical signs of all these conditions vary depending on those parts of the nervous system where the lesions are most severe. Commonly, however, the clinical picture is one of multifocal, asymmetric, intracranial disease seen in a young to middle-aged (or older) small-breed dog.

Case 7

Patient signalment

A 5-year-old female spayed yellow Labrador Retriever.

History

The dog was presented with a 1-year history of generalized seizures. She had three discrete seizures within the first 3 months after which time she was started on phenobarbital at 3 mg/kg PO q12h. CBC and serum biochemistry results were within normal limits. The seizures were described as tonic-clonic movements in lateral recumbence with salivation and urination at most episodes and occasional defecation. She was perceived to be unconscious during the events. Each seizure was noted to last approximately 2 min in duration. Her postictal phase lasted 10 min and was marked by ataxia and sedation. Monthly seizures for 6 months followed initiation of phenobarbital, therefore her phenobarbital dose was increased to 3.7 mg/kg PO q12h. The serum phenobarbital concentration was 28 µg/ml following this dose increase. No additional seizures were noted for 3 months. Two additional seizures within 30 days were noted, prompting referral for evaluation.

Physical examination

- **EENT:** No concerning abnormalities.
- **Lymph nodes:** No peripheral lymphadenopathy.
- **Oropharyngeal:** Normal.
- **Integument:** No concerning abnormalities.
- **Musculoskeletal:** No clinical abnormalities.
- **Abdominal palpation:** Soft, nonpainful palpation.
- **Urogenital:** Normal.
- **Respiratory:** No abnormalities detected.
- **Cardiac:** No abnormalities detected.

Neurologic examination

- **Mentation:** BAR.
- **Cranial nerve exam:** Normal.
- **Spinal reflexes:** Normal tone and spinal reflexes.
- **Postural reactions:** Paw replacement was normal in all four limbs. Hopping was normal in both thoracic limbs and not performed in either pelvic limb.
- **Gait assessment:** Ambulatory without evidence of paresis, ataxia, or lameness.
- **Spinal palpation:** No pain on palpation.
- **Cervical range of motion:** Normal.
- **Other:** None.

Neuroanatomic lesion localization practice sheet

Use this space below to work through NALL for Case 7. When you have finished, turn to the answer section on the following page to check your answers.

Abnormality	Possible NALL	Possible NALL	Possible NALL	Possible NALL	Possible NALL	Possible NALL

Discussion on neuroanatomic lesion localization

Abnormality	Possible NALL	Possible NALL	Possible NALL	Possible NALL	Possible NALL	Possible NALL
History of seizures	Prosencephalon/ forebrain					
No abnormalities noted on neurologic examination						

Neuroanatomic lesion localization, Case 7: Forebrain/prosencephalon

The neurologic examination was suggestive of a lesion affecting the forebrain. A dog or cat with a history of seizures should always have forebrain listed as a localization. All seizures originate from this region of the nervous system, regardless of underlying etiology. In this case, the dog also had a normal neurologic examination. Therefore, lateralization to the left or right forebrain is not possible. Furthermore, because no other neurologic abnormalities were noted, multifocal neurologic disease can also be ruled out.

Differential diagnoses

The differential diagnoses for a lesion causing seizures for 1 year, without evidence of neurological deficits interictal, would be a very short list. The history and examination strongly suggest idiopathic epilepsy. Idiopathic epilepsy is suspected to have a polygenic, recessive inheritance in Labrador Retriever dogs with onset time between 1 and 3 years of age. Therefore, idiopathic epilepsy would be a clear suspicion in this dog. Other differential diagnosis such as infectious or inflammatory meningoencephalitis, CVA, and neoplasia are less likely due to the chronicity of seizures, in the absence of neurologic examination abnormalities, prior to referral. Congenital brain disease, such as hydrocephalus, is expected to result in seizure development within the first 2 years of life and is therefore unlikely. No history of head trauma, in which the pet loses consciousness, was provided. Metabolic disease would be excluded based on a history of normal laboratory values.

Diagnostic testing and results

- **CBC:** No abnormalities.
- **Serum biochemistry:** No abnormalities.
- **Thoracic radiographs:** Normal.
- **MRI (brain):** Normal, no evidence of disease.

- **CSF analysis:** TNCC = 2 WBCs/µl (normal, < 5 cells/µl), protein = 13 µg/ml (normal, < 20 µg/ml), and no RBCs.
- **Serum phenobarbital concentration:** 28 µg/ml at a dosage of 3.7 mg/kg PO q12h.

Case conclusion

The dog was diagnosed with idiopathic epilepsy based on the history, normal neurologic examination, normal brain MRI, and normal CSF analysis. If we had also performed a bile acid test, this diagnosis would be considered a Tier II level diagnosis by the International Veterinary Epilepsy Task Force (De Risio *et al.*, 2015). The serum phenobarbital concentration was within the therapeutic range for a dog; however this serum concentration had been evaluated 4 months prior to referral (Bhatti *et al.*, 2015). The serum phenobarbital concentration was slightly reduced, at 25 µg/ml, and still within the canine reference range; however, a dose increase was recommended for improved seizure control (Bhatti *et al.*, 2015). Phenobarbital may have autoinduction in dogs, resulting a gradual reduction in serum concentration over time (Abramson, 1988); therefore the serum phenobarbital concentration was reevaluated and the phenobarbital dosage increased. Following the dose increase, the dog was seizure-free for 3 months before resuming seizures approximately every 3 months for several cycles.

Case 8

Patient signalment

A 10-year-old male neutered Husky.

History

The dog was presented with a 2-week history of progressive difficulty eating and change in voice. Prior to referral for a neurologic consultation, the primary veterinarian had performed a CBC, serum biochemistry and a T4, and no significant abnormalities were noted.

Physical examination

- **EENT:** No concerning abnormalities.
- **Lymph nodes:** No peripheral lymphadenopathy.
- **Oropharyngeal:** Evidence of tongue atrophy (see 'Neurologic examination' below) and dental disease.
- **Integument:** No concerning abnormalities.

- **Musculoskeletal:** Mild crepitus of stifles with reduced range of motion of the left stifle, otherwise normal.
- **Abdominal palpation:** Soft, nonpainful palpation.
- **Urogenital:** Normal.
- **Respiratory:** No abnormalities detected.
- **Cardiac:** No abnormalities detected.

Neurologic examination

- **Mentation:** Mildly obtunded.
- **Cranial nerve exam:** Unilateral right tongue atrophy with mild curvature to the right. Remainder of the cranial nerve examination was normal (Fig. 4.6).
- **Spinal reflexes:** Normal spinal reflexes.
- **Postural reactions:** Proprioceptive placing was reduced on the right thoracic and right pelvic limbs only.
- **Gait assessment:** Ambulatory with mild right hemiparesis, and lameness of the left pelvic limb.
- **Spinal palpation:** No pain on palpation of the neck and thoracolumbar spinal column.
- **Cervical range of motion:** Normal.
- **Other:** None.

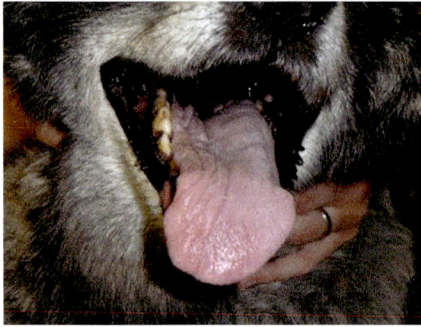

Fig. 4.6. Photo of the dog in Case 8 with unilateral right-sided tongue atrophy.

Neuroanatomic lesion localization practice sheet

Use this space below to work through NALL for Case 8. When you have finished, turn to the answer section on the following page to check your answers.

Abnormality	Possible NALL	Possible NALL	Possible NALL	Possible NALL	Possible NALL	Possible NALL

Discussion on neuroanatomic lesion localization

Abnormality	Possible NALL	Possible NALL	Possible NALL	Possible NALL	Possible NALL	Possible NALL
Obtunded	Forebrain/prosencephalon	Brainstem				
Tongue atrophy (right) with right deviation	CN XII, chronic (to cause deviation)					
Reduced right postural reactions	Forebrain/prosencephalon (left)	Brainstem (right)	C1–C5 myelopathy (right)	C6–T2 myelopathy (right)	Peripheral neuropathy	Neuromuscular junction

Neuroanatomic lesion localization, Case 8: Right brainstem, in the region of the nucleus for CN XII

The neurologic examination was suggestive of a lesion affecting the right brainstem. Change in mentation, including obtunded, stupor, or coma, may suggest brainstem and, less commonly, forebrain disease. The most helpful feature for neuroanatomic lesion localization in this case was the unilateral tongue atrophy and mild deviation. The paired nuclei for CN XII are located in the caudal aspect of the medulla, along the ventral aspect of the brainstem (de Lahunta and Glass, 2009). Innervation to the muscle of the tongue occurs via CN XII. Acute dysfunction of CN XII will result in unilateral flaccidity with deviation away from the side of the lesion due to intact function of the opposing side. Chronic denervation will result in visually apparent ipsilateral tongue atrophy and deviation toward the side of the lesion, due to contracture from muscle atrophy and fibrosis of the affected side. Unilateral tongue atrophy must involve the medulla, at the nucleus of CN XII, or the peripheral portion of CN XII. Signs of mentation changes, paw replacement deficits, and/or hemiparesis suggest brainstem involvement in this case. The proprioceptive pathways traverse rostrally from the spinal cord, through the medulla, to higher brainstem or forebrain centers. These paths may be disrupted by a lesion anywhere along the pathway, resulting in deficits. Motor tracts, conversely, pass from the higher motor centers in the forebrain and rostral brainstem caudally to synapse on LMNs in the spinal cord. These paths may also be disrupted by a lesion anywhere along the pathway, resulting in hemiparesis. Finally, mentation changes are noted when a lesion affecting the RAS in the brainstem is interrupted. A lesion affecting right ventral brainstem is likely to result in damage to CN XII, ipsilateral hemiparesis, mentation changes, and/or paw replacement deficits, as in this case.

Differential diagnoses

The differential diagnoses for a lesion for a chronic right brainstem lesion affecting the caudal ventral medulla include neoplasia (meningioma most commonly) and granuloma (infectious or inflammatory).

Diagnostic testing and results

- **CBC:** Unremarkable.
- **Serum biochemistry:** Unremarkable.
- **Thoracic radiographs:** Normal.
- **Abdominal ultrasonography:** No significant abnormalities.
- **MRI (brain):** A ventral, uniformly enhancing extra-axial mass was noted at the caudal ventral aspect of the caudal fossa causing deviation to the right of the caudal brainstem. Findings consistent with neoplasia, meningioma considered most likely.

Case conclusion

The dog was started on an anti-inflammatory dose of prednisone (1 mg/kg/day PO) due to the presence of suspected peritumoral edema. Radiation therapy was discussed with the clients and declined. Prednisone was continued for 14 days, then tapered to lowest effective dose to maintain the dog's quality of life. Instructions on monitoring food and water intake were provided, and a "meat ball" consistency of food was suggested because this was thought to be easiest for the dog to swallow with his tongue dysfunction. Humane euthanasia was elected 2 weeks after discharge, due to poor quality of life (Rossmeisl et al., 2013).

References

Abramson, F.P. (1988) Autoinduction of phenobarbital elimination in the dog. *Journal of Pharmaceutical Sciences* 77(9), 768–770. doi: 10.1002/jps.2600770910.

Bhatti, S.F.M., De Risio, L., Muñana, K., Penderis, J., Stein, V.M., et al. (2015) International Veterinary Epilepsy Task Force consensus proposal: medical treatment of canine epilepsy in Europe. *BMC Veterinary Research* 11(1), 176. doi: 10.1186/s12917-015-0464-z.

Bongartz, U., Nessler, J., Maiolini, A., Stein, V.M., Tipold, A. and Bathen-Nöthen, A. (2020) Vestibular disease in dogs: association between neurological examination, MRI lesion localisation and outcome. *The Journal of Small Animal Practice* 61(1), 57–64. doi: 10.1111/jsap.13070.

Cameron, S., Rishniw, M., Miller, A.D., Sturges, B. and Dewey, C.W. (2015) Characteristics and survival of 121 cats undergoing excision of intracranial meningiomas (1994–2011). *Veterinary Surgery* 44(6), 772–776. doi: 10.1111/vsu.12340.

Coates, J.R. and Jeffery, N.D. (2014) Perspectives on meningoencephalomyelitis of unknown origin. *Veterinary Clinics of North America: Small Animal Practice* 44(6), 1157–1185. doi: 10.1016/j.cvsm.2014.07.009.

Cornelis, I., Van Ham, L., Gielen, I., De Decker, S. and Bhatti, S.F.M. (2019) Clinical presentation, diagnostic findings, prognostic factors, treatment and outcome in dogs with meningoencephalomyelitis of unknown origin: a review. *Veterinary Journal* 244, 37–44.

de Lahunta, A. and Glass, E. (2009) *Veterinary Neuroanatomy and Clinical Neurology*, 3rd edn. Saunders Elsevier, St. Louis, Missouri.

De Risio, L., Bhatti, S., Muñana, K., Penderis, J., Stein, V., et al. (2015) International veterinary epilepsy task force consensus proposal: diagnostic approach to epilepsy in dogs. *BMC Veterinary Research* 11(1), 148. doi: 10.1186/s12917-015-0462-1.

Gradner, G., Kaefinger, R. and Dupre, G. (2019) Complications associated with ventriculoperitoneal shunts in dogs and cats with idiopathic hydrocephalus: a systematic review. *Journal of Veterinary Internal Medicine* 33(2), 403–412. doi: 10.1111/jvim.15422.

Hecht, S. and Adams, W.H. (2010) MRI of brain disease in veterinary patients part 1: basic principles and congenital brain disorders. *Veterinary Clinics of North America: Small Animal Practice* 40(1), 21–38. doi: 10.1016/j.cvsm.2009.09.005.

Korner, M., Roos, M., Meier, V.S., Soukup, A., Cancedda, S., et al. (2019) Radiation therapy for intracranial tumours in cats with neurological signs. *Journal of Feline Medicine and Surgery* 21(8), 765–771. doi: 10.1177/1098612X18801032.

Lamm, C.G. and Rezabeck, G.B. (2008) Parvovirus infection in domestic companion animals. *Veterinary Clinics of North America: Small Animal Practice* 38(4), 837–850. doi: 10.1016/j. cvsm.2008.03.008.

Lowrie, M. (2021) Guide to tremor and twitch syndromes in dogs and cats. *In Practice* 43(1), 4–17. doi: 10.1002/inpr.3.

Mikszewski, J.S. and Vite, C.H. (2005) Central nervous system dysfunction associated with Rocky Mountain spotted fever infection in five dogs. *Journal of the American Animal Hospital Association* 41(4), 259–266.

Penderis, J. (2009) The wobbly cat. Diagnostic and therapeutic approach to generalised ataxia. *Journal of Feline Medicine and Surgery* 11(5), 349–359.

Poncelet, L., Héraud, C., Springinsfeld, M., Ando, K., Kabova, A., *et al.* (2013) Identification of feline panleukopenia virus proteins expressed in Purkinje cell nuclei of cats with cerebellar hypoplasia. *Veterinary Journal* 196(3), 381–387. doi: 10.1016/j.tvjl.2012.10.019.

Rossmeisl, J.H. Jr, Jones, J.C., Zimmerman, K.L. and Robertson, J.L. (2013) Survival times following hospital discharge in dogs with palliatively treated primary brain tumors. *Journal of the American Veterinary Medical Association* 242(2), 193–198.

Schmidt, M.J., Hartmann, A., Farke, D., Failling, K. and Kolecka, M. (2019) Association between improvement of clinical signs and decrease of ventricular volume after ventriculoperitoneal shunting in dogs with internal hydrocephalus. *Journal of Veterinary Internal Medicine* 33(3), 1368–1375. doi: 10.1111/jvim.15468.

Stuetzer, B. and Hartmann, K. (2014) Feline parvovirus infection and associated diseases. *Veterinary Journal* 201(2), 150–155.

Van Asselt, N., Christensen, N., Meier, V., Rohrer Bley, C., Laliberte, S., *et al.* (2020) Definitive-intent intensity modulated radiation therapy provides similar outcomes to those previously published for definitive-intent three-dimensional conformal radiation therapy in dogs with primary brain tumors: a multi-institutional retrospective study. *Veterinary Radiology & Ultrasound* 61(4), 481–489.

5 Spinal Cord Disease

Susan Arnold[1], Heidi Barnes Heller[2]*, Joy Delamaide Gasper[3] and Julien Guevar[4]

[1]University of Minnesota, St. Paul, Minnesota, USA; [2]Barnes Veterinary Specialty Services, Madison, Wisconsin, USA; [3]Madison Veterinary Specialists, Madison, Wisconsin, USA; [4]University of Bern, Bern, Switzerland

Unless otherwise noted, all images and videos are owned by the lead author.

Case 1

Patient signalment

A 5-year-old male neutered Rhodesian Ridgeback mix.

History

Four days prior to presentation the dog was noted to limp on his right front leg. The following day he was still lame, and uncomfortable. The day before presentation he was noted to have progressive weakness in the right front leg and scuff the toe when walking. The dog was evaluated by a veterinarian, and the physical examination showed right thoracic limb weakness with subjectively reduced sensory responses in the toes. Radiographs of the cervical spine were unremarkable. Gabapentin (300 mg PO q12h) and carprofen (50 mg PO q12h) were prescribed.

Progression to involve the left thoracic limb was noted along with trembling when he tried to move. Inappropriate defecation was noted in the home as well as a reduced appetite.

*Email: barnes@barnesveterinaryservices.com

© CAB International 2022. *Small Animal Neuroanatomic Lesion Localization Practice Book*
(ed. H. Barnes Heller)
DOI: 10.1079/9781789247947.0005

Physical examination

T: 38.6°C/101.5°F   P: 160 beats/min   R: panting

- **EENT:** No concerning abnormalities.
- **Lymph nodes:** No peripheral lymphadenopathy.
- **Oropharyngeal:** No abnormalities noted.
- **Integument:** No ectoparasites seen.
- **Musculoskeletal:** No abnormalities noted.
- **Abdominal palpation:** Soft, no masses or ascites palpated.
- **Urogenital:** Urinary bladder large, not able to manually express.
- **Respiratory:** No abnormalities noted.
- **Cardiac:** No abnormalities noted.

Neurologic examination

- **Mentation:** Alert, responsive.
- **Cranial nerve exam:** All normal.
- **Spinal reflexes:** All normal.
- **Postural reactions:** Absent paw replacement in the right thoracic limb, reduced paw replacement in the left thoracic limb, and reduced paw replacement in both pelvic limbs.
- **Gait assessment:** Ambulatory tetraparesis with proprioceptive ataxia. His weakest limb was the right front with moderate paresis in the left front, and mild paraparesis. The right front leg may slide out in front or knuckle and slide under the patient's body. In lateral recumbency, his limbs were very stiff and tense, requiring withdrawal reflex testing to get him to bend his legs.
- **Spinal palpation:** Tense muscles on palpation, but no definitive location of pain.
- **Cervical range of motion:** Painful with neck range of motion.
- **Other:** None.

Neuroanatomic lesion localization practice sheet

Use this space below to work through NALL for Case 1. When you have finished, turn to the answer section on the following page to check your answers.

Abnormality	Possible NALL	Possible NALL	Possible NALL	Possible NALL	Possible NALL	Possible NALL

Discussion on neuroanatomic lesion localization

Abnormality	Possible NALL	Possible NALL	Possible NALL	Possible NALL	Possible NALL	Possible NALL
Reduced to absent paw replacement in all four limbs	Forebrain/prosencephalon	Brainstem	C1–C5 myelopathy	C6–T2 myelopathy	Peripheral neuropathy	Neuromuscular junction
Tetraparesis	Forebrain/prosencephalon	Brainstem	C1–C5 myelopathy	C6–T2 myelopathy	Peripheral neuropathy	Neuromuscular junction
Proprioceptive ataxia of all four limbs	Forebrain/prosencephalon	Brainstem	C1–C5 myelopathy			
Neck pain	C1–C5 myelopathy	C6–T2 myelopathy	Referred intracranial pain	Non-neurologic causes		
Increased tone in all four legs	Forebrain/prosencephalon	Brainstem	C1–C5 myelopathy			

Neuroanatomic lesion localization, Case 1: C1–C5 myelopathy

To start, it is important to first note that intracranial signs such as seizures, cranial nerve deficits, and cerebellar gait abnormalities are NOT noted. The lesion is not intracranial. Next, note that all four limbs are affected with the gait abnormalities and proprioceptive testing. This suggests either a C1–C5 or C6–T2 myelopathy or neuromuscular disease affecting all four limbs. Third, note that all reflexes were normal and there was increased tone. Animals with tetraparesis may have a neuromuscular localization, however the reflexes are expected to be reduced to absent in that situation and tone is usually reduced. When all four limbs are affected (tetraparesis), without evidence of neuromuscular disease, the lesion must be a C1–C5 or C6–T2 myelopathy. Normal thoracic limb reflexes reduce the likelihood of a C6–T2 myelopathy, therefore C1–C5 myelopathy was considered most likely in this dog. The profound degree of tetraparesis and ataxia, combined with neck pain, also leads to localization in the cervical spinal cord.

General proprioception is complex but important when localizing this dog's neurologic signs. All spinal nerves have general proprioceptive afferent neuron sensors in a receptor organ (muscle, tendon, joint). The axons course proximally in the limb via the appropriate spinal nerve, to the spinal cord. The cell body of that general proprioceptive afferent is in the segmental spinal (dorsal root) ganglion. The axon enters the spinal cord, and then the general proprioceptive axons concerned with conscious proprioception do not synapse but enter the dorsal funiculus (top part of the spinal cord white matter) and course cranially, for the most part in the fasciculus gracilis and faciculus cuneutus. Once in the midbrain these tracts cross to the contralateral cerebral cortex. Damage anywhere along this pathway (peripheral nerve, spinal cord, brainstem, or forebrain/prosencephalon) can result in proprioceptive deficits as shown in the paw replacement deficits in this dog (de Lahunta and Glass, 2009).

Differential diagnoses

The patient's history, NALL, and signalment resulted in the development of the following differential diagnoses: Intervertebral disc disease with intervertebral disc herniation, inflammatory/infectious meningomyelitis, discospondylitis, fracture or subluxation, or neoplasia.

Diagnostic testing and results

- **CBC:** No clinically significant abnormalities.
- **Chemistry panel:** No clinically significant abnormalities.
- **Canine SNAP 4Dx Plus panel:** Negative.
- **MRI (brain):** C3–C4 intervertebral disc herniation with ventrolateral compression and dorsolateral compression from hemorrhagic fat and hematoma. Multiple degenerative discs noted *in situ* with no clinical significance (Figs 5.1 and 5.2).

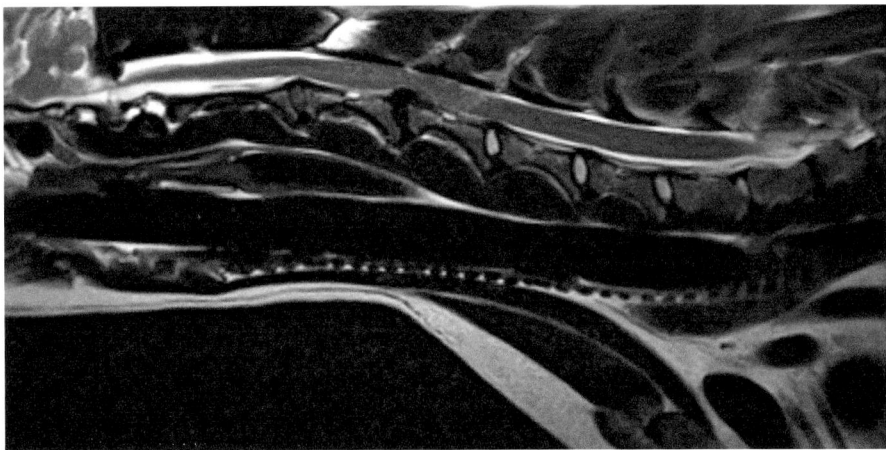

Fig. 5.1. T2W sagittal image of the cervical spinal cord in Case 1. Note the hypointense intervertebral disc at C3–C4 and the dorsal deviation of the spinal cord. (Image used with permission from Dr. Joy Delamaide Gasper.)

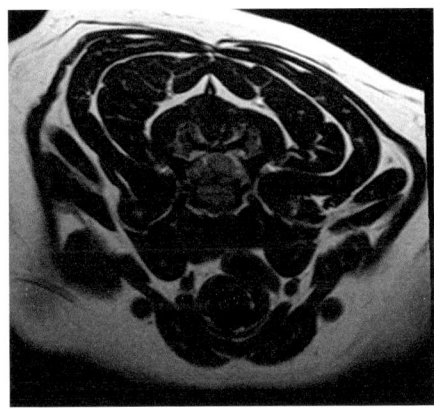

Fig. 5.2. T2W transverse image at the level of C3–C4 in Case 1. Note the right ventral compression causing right C4 nerve root compression and mild ventral spinal cord compression. Findings are consistent with an intervertebral disc extrusion with hemorrhage and nerve root compression. (Image used with permission from Dr. Joy Delamaide Gasper.)

Case conclusion

- **Procedure:** Right C3–C4 hemilaminectomy with dorsal cervical approach.

Most patients that have a cervical disc herniation can be treated with a ventral approach in order to perform a ventral slot surgery (Sharp and Wheeler, 2004). However, in this patient's case, the compression was too far lateralized, and extended too far along the length of the vertebral body, to be adequately decompressed from a ventral slot. This approach involves a much thicker layer of muscle dissection and can take a longer postoperative hospitalization to recover. A hemilaminectomy was made, which allowed adequate access to remove a large amount of disc material mixed with hematoma and fat from the side of the spinal cord as well as a large amount of mineralized disc material from under the spinal cord.

This patient initially recovered well. At the 2-week recheck examination, he was ambulatory with mild right front leg monoparesis and proprioceptive ataxia in all four limbs. He had absent paw replacement in the right front leg, reduced in the right rear leg, and normal paw replacement on the left. Unfortunately, this patient was presented again at a 6-week recheck for recurrence of severe persistent neck pain despite regaining strength and coordination. A second MRI was performed, which showed persistent/recurrent disc material under the spinal cord at the level of C3–C4. A ventral slot surgery was recommended to relieve this spinal cord compression. However, the family declined surgery and the dog was euthanized. This is an atypical situation, as most patients that have surgery for an acute intervertebral disc herniation can make a complete and often long-lasting recovery.

Case 2

Patient signalment

An 11-year-old female spayed Labrador Retriever.

History

Three weeks prior to presentation, the dog demonstrated reduced activity, did not wag her tail as expected, and discontinued playing with other dogs in the house. When posturing to defecate, she would not hold her tail out away from her body and appeared painful in her low back. No fecal or urinary incontinence was noted. Lateral radiographs of her neck and back showed narrowed disc spaces at C2–C3 and T13–L1. She was presented on carprofen (50 mg PO q12h) and gabapentin (300 mg PO q8–12h), which seemed to improve her mobility and comfort.

Physical examination

T: 38.5°C/101.4°F   P: 120 beats/min   R: panting

- **EENT:** No concerning abnormalities.
- **Lymph nodes:** No peripheral lymphadenopathy.
- **Oropharyngeal:** Normal.
- **Integument:** No ectoparasites seen.
- **Musculoskeletal:** Stifles severe bilateral medial buttress, mild bilateral hind limb muscle atrophy.
- **Abdominal palpation:** Soft, no masses or ascites palpated.
- **Urogenital:** No concerning abnormalities.
- **Respiratory**: Normal.
- **Cardiac:** No abnormalities noted.

Neurologic examination

- **Mentation:** Alert, responsive.
- **Cranial nerve exam:** All normal.
- **Spinal reflexes:** All normal.
- **Postural reactions:** Absent paw replacement on both pelvic limbs, normal paw replacement on both thoracic limbs.
- **Gait assessment:** Ambulatory, mild paraparesis and proprioceptive ataxia.
- **Spinal palpation:** Tense with cervical palpation, remainder nonpainful.
- **Cervical range of motion:** Normal.
- **Other:** Dropped flaccid, paretic tail.

Neuroanatomic lesion localization practice sheet

Use this space below to work through NALL for Case 2. When you have finished, turn to the answer section on the following page to check your answers.

Abnormality	Possible NALL	Possible NALL	Possible NALL	Possible NALL	Possible NALL	Possible NALL

Discussion on neuroanatomic lesion localization

Abnormality	Possible NALL	Possible NALL	Possible NALL	Possible NALL	Possible NALL	Possible NALL	Possible NALL	Possible NALL
Reduced to absent paw replacement testing in pelvic limbs	Forebrain/prosencephalon	Brainstem	C1–C5 myelopathy	C6–T2 myelopathy	T3–L3 myelopathy	L4–S3 myelopathy/radiculopathy	Peripheral neuropathy	Neuromuscular junction
Paraparesis	T3–L3 myelopathy	L4–S3 myelopathy/radiculopathy	Peripheral neuropathy	Neuromuscular junction	Myopathy			
Proprioceptive ataxia of pelvic limbs	C6–T2 myelopathy	T3–L3 myelopathy						
Neck pain	C1–C5 myelopathy	C6–T2 myelopathy	Referred intracranial pain	Non-neurologic causes				
Flaccid tail	S1–S3	Coccygeal muscles						

Neuroanatomic lesion localization, Case 2: Cauda equina syndrome/L6–S3 radiculopathy

To start, it is important to first note that intracranial signs such as seizures, cranial nerve deficits, and cerebellar gait abnormalities are NOT noted. The lesion is not intracranial. Next, note that only the pelvic limbs are affected along with the tail. These findings should focus your attention caudal to T2 spinal cord segment. Normal pelvic limb reflexes could suggest a T3–L3 myelopathy; however, that is not the case with this dog. There is an occasional case, like this one, where tail paresis is the best indicator of NALL. Innervation to tail function arises at the L7–S3 nerve roots, therefore the lesion must involve one of these segments. In this case, the patient's gait was mildly affected, due to the integrity of the majority of the lumbosacral intumescence, associated nerve roots, and remaining spinal cord cranial to L6. The paw replacement deficits may have been associated with subclinical sciatic nerve dysfunction. In subtle or early sciatic nerve involvement, paresis or paw replacement deficits may be noted prior to the onset of reflex deficits. The tail paresis suggests this may be the case. Changes in her ability to voluntarily defecate also indicated that the problem was in the lumbosacral region (Granger *et al.*, 2020).

Differential diagnoses

Intervertebral disc herniation, neoplasia, and inflammatory or infectious neuritis.

Diagnostic testing and results

- **CBC:** No clinically significant abnormalities (testing performed at primary veterinary clinic).
- **Biochemistry panel:** No clinically significant abnormalities (testing performed at primary veterinary clinic).
- **MRI (lumbosacral region):** Intraparenchymal T2W and STIR hyperintense lesion at level of L5 was noted. The most likely cause was neoplasia, however inflammatory or infectious myelitis could not be eliminated (Figs 5.3 and 5.4).
- **CSF analysis:** Unable to obtain fluid.

Case conclusion

Intramedullary spinal cord tumors are rare. Ependymomas are the most common and gliomas (astrocytoma, oligodendroglioma) are the second most common. Ependymal cell tumors are more uniformly contrast-enhancing, compared to glial cell tumors, therefore this was most likely glial cell in origin (Pancotto

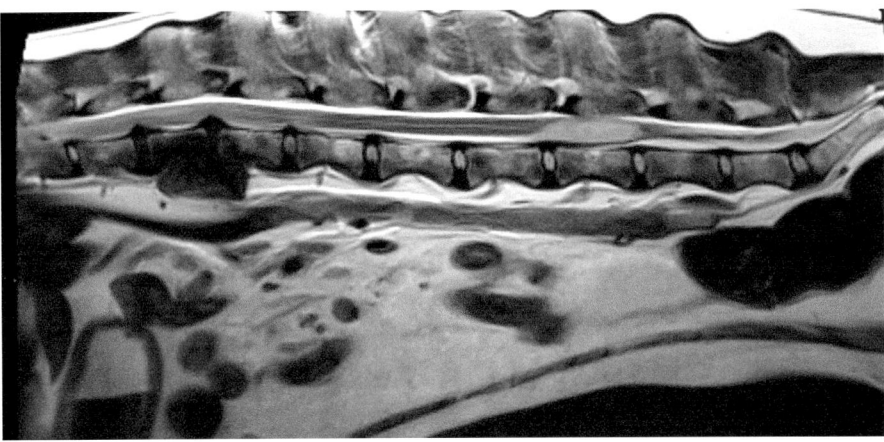

Fig. 5.3. T2W sagittal image of the lumbar spine in Case 2. A hyperintense lesion is noted extending from the caudal body of L4 caudally to the L5–L6 intervertebral disc space. (Image used with permission from Dr. Joy Delamaide Gasper.)

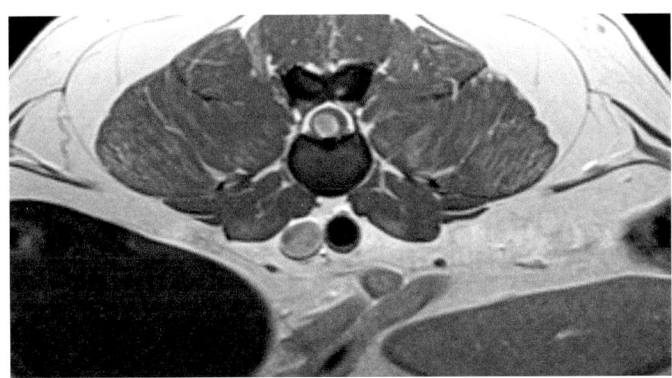

Fig. 5.4. T1W post-contrast transverse image at mid-body of L5 in Case 2. Contrast-enhancing intramedullary mass is noted in the spinal cord. (Image used with permission from Dr. Joy Delamaide Gasper.)

et al., 2013). Radiation therapy was recommended along with prednisone for anti-inflammatory and anti-edema effects.

The dog was treated with stereotactic radiosurgery radiation therapy with three doses of 8 Gy each. At the 2-month recheck examination the dog was ambulatory with mild pelvic limb weakness and ataxia. She had regained the ability to wag her tail but had persistent reduced paw replacement in the pelvic limbs. Perineal reflex remained absent but appeared to have normal anal tone and was nonpainful. The client reported she had improved ability to control defecation.

Case 3

Patient signalment

A 7-year female spayed Labrador Retriever mix.

History

For approximately 1 year, the dog demonstrated a gradual reduction in normal activity including difficulty jumping in and out of the truck and walking more slowly when walking. Sporadic yelping was noted, which occurred occasionally when touched on the lumbar region. When walking, scuffing was noted in the pelvic limbs. Recently, the dog had a reduced appetite.

She was evaluated by a board-certified surgeon, who described that her back legs would take two steps for every one step in the front. Tramadol (50 mg PO q8h) and gabapentin (200 mg PO q8h) were prescribed; however no improvement was noted.

Physical examination

T: 39.2°C/102.5°F   P: 140 beats/min   R: panting

- **EENT:** No concerning abnormalities.
- **Lymph nodes:** No peripheral lymphadenopathy.
- **Oropharyngeal:** No concerning abnormalities.
- **Integument:** No abnormalities noted.
- **Musculoskeletal:** No abnormalities noted.
- **Abdominal palpation:** Soft, nonpainful, no palpable masses.
- **Urogenital:** No abnormalities noted.
- **Respiratory:** No abnormalities noted.
- **Cardiac:** No abnormalities noted.

Neurologic examination

- **Mentation:** Alert.
- **Cranial nerve exam:** All normal.
- **Spinal reflexes:** Withdrawal reflexes normal in all limbs, bicep reflexes normal bilaterally, patellar reflexes increased bilaterally, cutaneous trunci reflex absent caudal to T8, remainder normal.

- **Postural reactions:** Bilateral absent paw replacement in the pelvic limbs, bilateral normal paw replacement in thoracic limbs.
- **Gait assessment:** Ambulatory, moderate paraparesis and proprioceptive ataxia, with a short and choppy gait in the front legs.
- **Spinal palpation:** Tense epaxial muscles from mid-neck to mid-thoracic region.
- **Cervical range of motion:** Head held low and unwilling to rotate head laterally left or right.
- **Other:** None.

Neuroanatomic lesion localization practice sheet

Use this space below to work through NALL for Case 3. When you have finished, turn to the answer section on the following page to check your answers.

Abnormality	Possible NALL	Possible NALL	Possible NALL	Possible NALL	Possible NALL	Possible NALL

Discussion on neuroanatomic lesion localization

Abnormality	Possible NALL	Possible NALL	Possible NALL	Possible NALL	Possible NALL	Possible NALL	Possible NALL	Possible NALL
Reduced to absent paw replacement in pelvic limbs	Forebrain/ prosencephalon	Brainstem	C1–C5 myelopathy	C6–T2 myelopathy	T3–L3 myelopathy	L4–S3 myelopathy/ radiculopathy	Peripheral neuropathy	Neuromuscular junction
Paraparesis	T3–L3 myelopathy	L4–S3 myelopathy/ radiculopathy	Peripheral neuropathy	Neuromuscular junction	Myopathy			
Proprioceptive ataxia of only pelvic limbs	C6–T2 myelopathy	T3–L3 myelopathy						
Two-engine gait (short choppy in thoracic limbs)	C6–T2 myelopathy							
Reduced cutaneous trunci reflex	T3–L3 myelopathy	Cutaneous sensory nerves	Lateral thoracic nerve	Panniculus muscle				
Increased patellar reflexes	C1–C5 myelopathy	C6–T2 myelopathy	T3–L3 myelopathy					
Neck pain	C1–C5 myelopathy	C6–T2 myelopathy	Referred intracranial pain	Non-neurologic causes				

Neuroanatomic lesion localization, Case 3: T3–L3 myelopathy, with a focus in the cranial thoracic spinal cord region

To start, identify that intracranial signs such as seizures, cranial nerve deficits, and cerebellar gait abnormalities are NOT noted. The lesion is not intracranial. Next, note that the pelvic limbs are demonstrating the majority of the abnormalities, but a gait abnormality was noted in the thoracic limbs. The most useful neurologic examination abnormalities are the character of the gait and the cutaneous trunci abnormality. This patient has a "two-engine gait", which refers to the appearance of the front legs moving at a different pace than the rear limbs. The front legs move in a short stride, stilted movement, compared to a floating, proprioceptive ataxia gait of the pelvic limbs. This gait abnormality typically indicates a low cervical or high thoracic lesion (De Decker *et al.*, 2012).

The cutaneous trunci reflex is a spinal reflex in which the afferent pathway is from a cutaneous sensory nerve which ascends up the spinal cord, then synapses on the lateral thoracic nerve (arising from C8–T1), which stimulates the panniculus muscle to contract. The reflex should be present from T2–T3 to the iliac crest, which is L6 for most dogs. Stimulation of the truncal dermatomes on one side results in twitching of the skin on the lateral aspect of the thorax bilaterally. Lesions result in a loss of the reflex one or two segments caudal to the site of the lesion. This patient's cutaneous trunci reflex was absent caudal to T8, which indicates that the spinal cord lesion is likely to be at T6 or T7.

Differential diagnoses

The patient's history, NALL, and signalment were accounted for when considering the differential diagnoses list. Although intervertebral disc herniation is common in the T3–L3 spinal cord region, it is uncommon cranial to T10. Neoplasia would be more likely cranial to T10. Additional differential diagnoses include infectious or inflammatory meningomyelitis and discospondylitis.

Diagnostic testing and results

- **CBC:** No significant abnormalities.
- **Serum biochemistry:** No significant abnormalities.
- **Total T4:** Results within normal range.
- **Canine SNAP 4Dx Plus panel:** Negative results.
- **Three-view thoracic radiographs:** No concerning abnormalities.
- **MRI (T3–L3 region):** Right T7 extradural mass—most consistent with meningioma, malignant peripheral nerve sheath tumor, or lymphoma (Fig. 5.5).
- **CSF (lumbar):** Unable to obtain fluid.

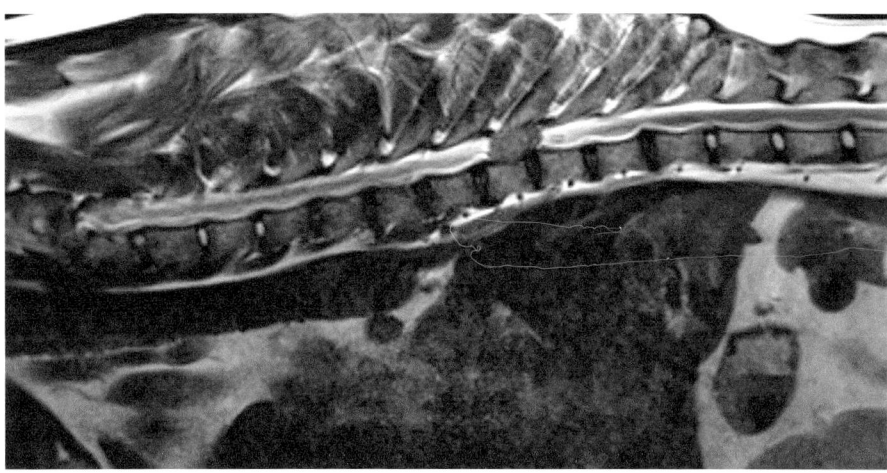

Fig. 5.5. T2W off-midline sagittal image of the thoracic spine in Case 3. A hypointense to spinal cord, isointense to bone lesion is noted at T7. (Image used with permission from Dr. Joy Delamaide Gasper.)

Case conclusion

In some dogs, surgical debulking can result in profound improvement in the neurologic signs (Pancotto *et al.*, 2013). Surgical biopsy can help to determine a more definitive diagnosis as well. Following surgery with radiation therapy provides a longer time of remission and is therefore recommended for many dogs. The owners of this dog did not elect to pursue surgical debulking, or radiation therapy. Therefore, prednisone was started to decrease swelling and inflammation around the suspected mass. Modest improvement was noted initially; however progressive worsening was again noted several weeks into treatment, therefore humane euthanasia was elected.

Case 4

Patient signalment

A 3-year-old female spayed mixed-breed dog.

History

The dog was presented for an acute onset of neck pain following a fall from the owner's bed. The dog did not have a history of prior medical disease.

Physical examination

T: Did not assess   P: Did not assess   R: panting

- **EENT:** No abnormalities noted.
- **Lymph nodes:** Normal, no peripheral lymphadenopathy appreciated.
- **Oropharyngeal:** No abnormalities noted.
- **Integument:** No abnormalities noted.
- **Musculoskeletal:** No abnormalities noted; however a full orthopedic examination was not performed.
- **Abdominal palpation:** Normal, soft, nonpainful, no masses or organomegaly appreciated.
- **Urogenital:** Normal external genitalia.
- **Respiratory:** No abnormalities noted.
- **Cardiac:** No murmurs or arrythmia noted.

Neurologic examination

- **Mentation:** Bright and alert.
- **Cranial nerve exam:** All cranial nerves were normal.
- **Spinal reflexes:** All spinal reflexes were normal.
- **Postural reactions:** Delayed paw replacement and hopping on all four legs.
- **Gait assessment:** Mild to moderate ambulatory tetraparesis.
- **Spinal palpation:** Pain on palpation of the neck.
- **Cervical range of motion:** Not performed due to the presence of spinal hyperesthesia on spinal palpation.
- **Other:** Low head carriage.

Neuroanatomic lesion localization practice sheet

Use this space below to work through NALL for Case 4. When you have finished, turn to the answer section on the following page to check your answers.

Abnormality	Possible NALL	Possible NALL	Possible NALL	Possible NALL	Possible NALL	Possible NALL

Discussion on neuroanatomic lesion localization

Abnormality	Possible NALL	Possible NALL	Possible NALL	Possible NALL	Possible NALL	Possible NALL
Tetraparesis	Prosencephalon (rare)	Brainstem	C1–C5 myelopathy	C6–T2 myelopathy	Peripheral neuropathy	Neuromuscular junction
Ataxia in all four limbs	Prosencephalon/ forebrain	Brainstem	C1–C5 myelopathy			
Delayed paw replacement all limbs	Prosencephalon (rare)	Brainstem	C1–C5 myelopathy	C6–T2 myelopathy	Peripheral neuropathy	Neuromuscular junction
Cervical pain on palpation	C1–C5 myelopathy	C6–T2 myelopathy	Referred intracranial disease	Non neurologic causes		

Neuroanatomic lesion localization, Case 4: C1–C5 myelopathy

Begin by identifying a lack of signs of intracranial disease including seizures, cranial nerve deficits, mentation changes, or cerebellar gait abnormalities. The lesion is not intracranial in this dog. Normal reflexes were identified, therefore neuromuscular disease is unlikely. Although a myopathy may cause paraparesis with normal reflexes, that was ruled out due to identification of paw replacement deficits in all four limbs. At this point, it would be reasonable to consider a spinal cord lesion localization. Evidence of tetraparesis with proprioceptive ataxia and reduced proprioceptive placing in all four limbs suggests the lesion is cranial to T2. If the lesion were caudal to T2, the thoracic limbs would not be affected. Therefore, the NALL was determined to be between C1 and T2. However, we can further narrow the localization in this dog based on the normal thoracic limb reflexes. Normal thoracic limb reflexes suggest the C6–T2 intumesces is intact and therefore a C1–C5 myelopathy is most likely.

Differential diagnoses

Acute onset signs localized to the cervical spine in a small-breed dog would suggest subluxation, fracture, or acute type I disc herniation. Other differential diagnoses include ANNPF and meningomyelitis if we consider the possibility that the dog fell as a result of neurologic disease rather than the fall resulting in neurologic disease.

Diagnostic testing and results

- **CBC:** Unremarkable.
- **Serum biochemistry:** No clinically significant abnormalities.
- **CT:** Acute, traumatic, mildly displaced C1 fracture with mild vertebral canal narrowing and spinal cord compression. Consider incomplete ossification of neural arch as predisposing/complicating factor (Fig. 5.6).

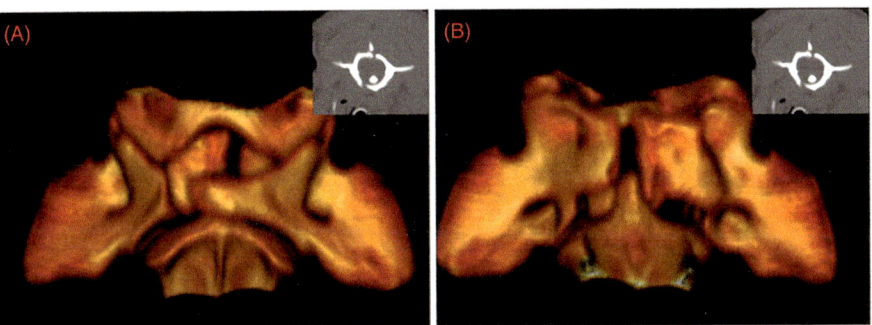

Fig. 5.6. Ventral view (A) and dorsal view (B) 3D reconstruction CT of Case 4 showing acute, traumatic, mildly displaced C1 fracture with mild vertebral canal narrowing and spinal cord compression. Consider incomplete ossification of neural arch as predisposing/complicating factor (Images used with permission from Dr. Julien Guevar.)

Case conclusion

The dog was suspected to have a preexisting, congenital, incomplete ossification of the atlas which had become unstable following the trauma (Warren-Smith *et al.*, 2009). The atlas was burst on to the midline into two hemi-atlases and the instability was responsible for the pain and the tetraparesis.

Surgical stabilization was recommended, and a soft cast was applied around the neck from the middle of the dog's head to the middle of her thorax to reduce cervical flexion during presurgical planning. Following surgical planning, three-dimensionally printed drill guides were designed to increase the safety of the surgery.

A ventral approach was performed, and stabilization was with screws and PMMA. No intraoperative complications were encountered, and she was discharged 3 days after surgery (Rodiño-Tilve *et al.*, 2017).

Incomplete ossification of the atlas, which may be associated with atlanto-axial subluxation, should be considered in the differential diagnosis of dogs with clinical signs localized to the cranial cervical region. Bone edges are often smooth and rounded with a superficial layer of relatively compact cortical bone. Osseous defects correspond to normal positions of sutures between the halves of the neural arch and the intercentrum and are therefore compatible with incomplete ossification of the atlas.

Case 5

Patient signalment

A 1-year-old spayed female Chihuahua.

History

The dog was presented for evaluation of pelvic limb weakness that was static over the past 6 months. She was adopted at 5 months of age and had never walked normally. At home, she walked with a stiff, uncoordinated gait with occasional scuffing of thoracic limb toes when walking. Collapse in all four limbs when walking was occasionally noted. She is up to date on vaccinations. She has not received any medications for her gait abnormalities. She eats a commercial puppy food and has not traveled anywhere recently, although her history prior to her adoption is unknown.

Physical examination

T: 39.1°C/102.4°F   P: 200 beats/min   R: 32 breaths/min

- **EENT:** No concerning abnormalities.
- **Lymph nodes:** No peripheral lymphadenopathy.

- **Oropharyngeal:** Normal.
- **Integument:** No concerning abnormalities.
- **Musculoskeletal:** No clinical abnormalities.
- **Abdominal palpation:** Soft, nonpainful palpation.
- **Urogenital:** Normal.
- **Respiratory:** No abnormalities detected.
- **Cardiac:** No abnormalities detected.

Neurologic examination

- **Mentation:** BAR.
- **Cranial nerve exam:** Normal.
- **Spinal reflexes:** Normal in all limbs; normal perianal reflex; normal cutaneous trunci reflex.
- **Postural reactions:** Delayed to absent paw replacement and hopping in all four limbs. Pelvic limb postural reaction deficits are more delayed than thoracic limb postural reaction deficits.
- **Gait assessment:** Ambulatory with mild tetraparesis and general proprioceptive ataxia of all limbs. Paresis and ataxia are more pronounced in the pelvic limbs compared to the thoracic limbs. The gait looks spastic with minimal flexion observed throughout the joints.
- **Spinal palpation:** No overt pain on palpation.
- **Cervical range of motion:** Not assessed.
- **Other:** Increased tone in all four limbs in recumbence. Very difficult to elicit withdrawal reflexes in the thoracic and pelvic limbs due to increased extensor rigidity.

Neuroanatomic lesion localization practice sheet

Use this space below to work through NALL for Case 5. When you have finished, turn to the answer section on the following page to check your answers.

Abnormality	Possible NALL	Possible NALL	Possible NALL	Possible NALL	Possible NALL	Possible NALL

Discussion on neuroanatomic lesion localization

Abnormality	Possible NALL	Possible NALL	Possible NALL	Possible NALL	Possible NALL	Possible NALL	Possible NALL
Tetraparesis	Forebrain/prosencephalon	Brainstem	C1–C5 myelopathy	C6–T2 myelopathy	Peripheral neuropathy	Neuromuscular junction	Myopathy
Proprioceptive ataxia all four limbs	Forebrain/prosencephalon	Brainstem	C1–C5 myelopathy				
Reduced to absent paw replacement	Forebrain/prosencephalon	Brainstem	C1–C5 myelopathy	C6–T2 myelopathy	Peripheral neuropathy	Neuromuscular junction	
Extensor rigidity all limbs	Forebrain/prosencephalon	Brainstem	C1–C5 myelopathy				

Neuroanatomic lesion localization, Case 5: C1–C5 myelopathy

To begin, note that this dog does not have signs of intracranial disease such as seizures, cranial nerve deficits, or cerebellar gait abnormalities. Therefore, this lesion is NOT intracranial. In patients with gait dysfunction in all four limbs, possible spinal cord NALL include the C1–C5 and C6–T2 regions of the spinal cord, and diffuse neuromuscular dysfunction. Patients with diffuse neuromuscular dysfunction are tetraparetic, but their tetraparesis is considered an "LMN" tetraparesis. This will lead to a short and choppy gait, so patients with diffuse neuromuscular disease look weak. This dog does not have a short, choppy gait, but instead looks stiff. Additionally, patients with diffuse neuromuscular disease do not develop a general proprioceptive ataxia. For these reasons, a diffuse neuromuscular cause of this dog's neurologic dysfunction is ruled out. A lesion in the C6–T2 region of the spinal cord manifests as weakness in the thoracic limbs, taking short, choppy steps, with decreased tone and decreased reflexes in the thoracic limbs. The reflexes in this patient were normal, therefore the lesion is NOT in the C6–T2 region of the spinal cord.

A lesion in the C1–C5 region of the spinal cord explains this dog's neurologic signs. Patients with C1–C5 myelopathies have UMN dysfunction in all four limbs. Due to loss of UMNs from both the pyramidal and extrapyramidal tracts, the LMNs innervating the limbs are freed from their UMN inhibition. This results in UMN paresis, which is characterized by spastic paresis or paralysis and increased muscle tone. Because the LMNs are not the site of the lesion, patients with C1–C5 myelopathies have normal thoracic and pelvic limb spinal reflexes. Postural reaction deficits occur due to disruption of ascending sensory projections that are involved in providing information about touch, pressure, and joint proprioception. Projections travel cranially through the spinal cord to the brain. Lesions in the spinal cord prevent sensory information from being carried to the brain. This results in postural reaction deficits and is also responsible for general proprioceptive ataxia. Based on the combination of UMN tetraparesis with general proprioceptive ataxia, increased muscle tone, and normal reflexes in all four limbs, and normal mentation and cranial nerves, the NALL is the C1–C5 region of this patient's spinal cord.

Range of motion was not performed due to the risk of subluxation of C1–C2 in this breed and age of dog.

Diagnostic testing and results

- **CBC:** Normal.
- **Blood chemistry panel:** Normal.
- **Cervical vertebral column radiographs:** Ventrodorsal and lateral views were obtained. On the lateral view, an increased distance is observed between the dorsal arch of C1 and the spinous process of C2. On the ventrodorsal view, no dens is visible, and subluxation of the C1–C2 joint is apparent. The final diagnosis was a subluxation of C1 and C2, also termed an atlantoaxial subluxation due to congenital malformation (Fig. 5.7).

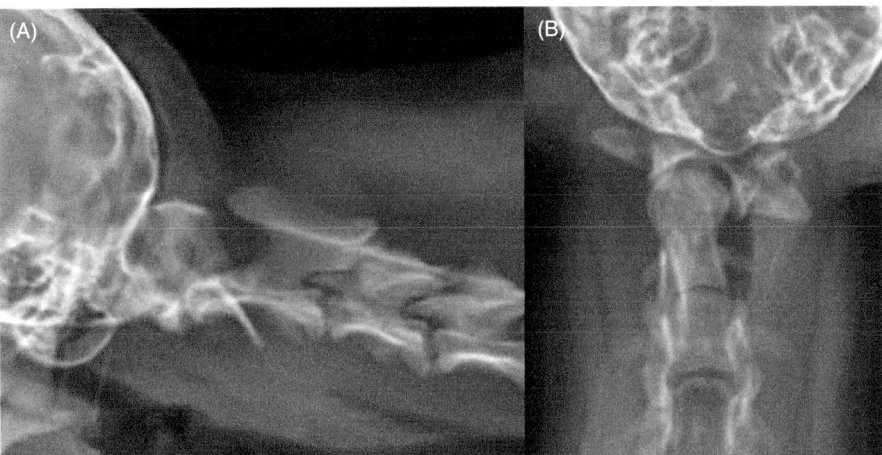

Fig. 5.7. Lateral and ventrodorsal radiographs of Case 5. On the lateral view (A), there is increased distance between the dorsal arch of C1 and the spinous process of C2. On the ventrodorsal view (B), a dens is not visible and subluxation of the C1–C2 joint is apparent. (Images used with permission from Dr. Susan Arnold.)

Case conclusion

Treatment options for an atlantoaxial subluxation consisted of surgical fixation or temporary cervical splinting (Havig *et al.*, 2005; Slanina, 2016). The owners elected to pursue surgical fixation. Surgery consisted of a ventral approach to the C1–C2 joint. Screws were placed into the ventral arch of C1 and the body of C2. The exposed screw heads were embedded in PMMA to hold the C1–C2 joint in rigid fixation. Recovery was uneventful over 8 weeks of postoperative restricted activity. The dog returned to a normal neurologic examination at the 8-week recheck and continued to be normal until 2 years of age, at which point she was lost to follow-up.

Case 6

Patient signalment

A 6-year-old neutered male Miniature Schnauzer.

History

The dog was presented for a peracute onset of difficulty using his pelvic limbs. He went for a walk the afternoon prior to presentation and seemed normal on this walk. That evening he was let outside, the owners heard a yelp, and found him unable to rise in the pelvic limbs. When he was assisted to stand, his owners noticed that his left pelvic limb seemed more affected than the right pelvic limb. The dog has a history of spending time unsupervised in the yard, which is encircled by an electric fence.

Historically, he had a urolith that was successfully treated with a dissolution diet and was attacked by another dog in the household 2 years prior. No residual injuries have been noted. He is up to date on vaccines and is not on any medications. He has not traveled anywhere. He eats a urinary dissolution kibble.

Physical examination

T: 38.6°C/101.5°F   P: 100 beats/min   R: panting

- **EENT:** Normal.
- **Lymph nodes:** Soft, small, symmetrical.
- **Oropharyngeal:** Moderate generalized dental disease; mucous membranes pink and moist; CRT < 2 s.
- **Integument:** Normal.
- **Musculoskeletal:** Normal.
- **Abdominal palpation:** Soft and nonpainful on palpation; no free fluid, masses, or organomegaly noted; bladder moderately distended.
- **Urogenital:** Normal external genitalia.
- **Respiratory:** Normal.
- **Cardiac:** No abnormalities detected.

Neurologic examination

- **Mentation:** BAR.
- **Cranial nerve exam:** Normal.
- **Spinal reflexes:** Normal.
- **Postural reactions:** Absent paw replacement and hopping in the left pelvic limb; absent paw replacement and moderately delayed hopping in the right pelvic limb; normal postural reactions in the thoracic limbs.
- **Gait assessment:** Nonambulatory with plegia in the left pelvic limb, and moderate paresis and general proprioceptive ataxia in the right pelvic limb.
- **Spinal palpation:** No pain on palpation.
- **Cervical range of motion:** Normal.
- **Other:** Increased extensor tone in both pelvic limbs, more pronounced in the left pelvic limb; nociception positive in the left pelvic limb.

Neuroanatomic lesion localization practice sheet

Use this space below to work through NALL for Case 6. When you have finished, turn to the answer section on the following page to check your answers.

Abnormality	Possible NALL	Possible NALL	Possible NALL	Possible NALL	Possible NALL	Possible NALL	Possible NALL

Discussion on neuroanatomic lesion localization

Abnormality	Possible NALL	Possible NALL	Possible NALL	Possible NALL	Possible NALL	Possible NALL
Monoplegia left pelvic limb, monoparesis right pelvic limb	Forebrain/ prosencephalon	Brainstem	C1–C5 myelopathy	C6–T2 myelopathy	Peripheral neuropathy	Neuromuscular junction
Delayed postural reactions	Forebrain/ prosencephalon	Brainstem	C1–C5 myelopathy	C6–T2 myelopathy	Peripheral neuropathy	Neuromuscular junction
Increased extensor tone in both pelvic limbs	T3–L3 myelopathy					

Neuroanatomic lesion localization, Case 6: T3–L3 myelopathy

To start, note that this dog does not have a history of seizures, or evidence of cranial nerve deficits, mentation changes, or cerebellar gait abnormalities. Therefore, the lesion is NOT intracranial. In patients with dysfunction of their pelvic limbs only, lesions affecting the C1–C5 and C6–T2 regions of the spinal cord can be eliminated. Patients with lesions affecting either the L4–S3 region of the spinal cord or the neuromuscular system of the pelvic limbs will have LMN dysfunction reflected as flaccid paresis/paralysis and/or reduced spinal reflexes in the pelvic limbs. The dog in this case did not have evidence of flaccid paresis or reduced reflexes, therefore a T3–L3 myelopathy is the likely NALL.

In a T3–L3 myelopathy, patients display UMN paraparesis and pelvic limb general proprioceptive ataxia. Paraparesis results from loss of UMNs, which travel caudally from the brain, through the spinal cord, to synapse with the LMNs that are found in the ventral horn of the spinal cord. These UMNs are responsible for initiating voluntary movement. Because these UMNs are inhibitory to the LMNs they synapse with, loss of UMNs leads to an increase in activity from the LMNs. In effect, UMN paraparesis leads to a stiffness rather than an overt weakness. Patients with UMN paresis take long, exaggerated steps due to lack of flexion. They have increased extensor tone in their limbs. Because a lesion in the T3–L3 region of the spinal cord does not affect pelvic limb reflex arcs, the pelvic limb reflexes are normal (not decreased) in a patient with a T3–L3 myelopathy. General proprioceptive ataxia, characterized by knuckling and crossing over midline during gait evaluation, and postural reaction deficits result from disruption of ascending sensory projections traveling from the pelvic limbs to the cerebral cortex (and the cerebellum for proprioception). The combination of UMN paraparesis, general proprioceptive ataxia, increased pelvic limb extensor tone, and normal pelvic limb spinal reflexes is consistent with a T3–L3 myelopathy.

Differential diagnoses

The peracute signs are most consistent with an FCEM. However, acute disc herniation, meningomyelitis, fracture or subluxation, or acute hemorrhage associated with neoplasia cannot be ruled out.

Diagnostic testing and results

- **CBC:** Normal.
- **Blood chemistry panel:** Normal.
- **Thoracolumbar MRI:** Moderate, predominately left-sided, intraparenchymal T2W hyperintensity of the spinal cord is present, extending from the level of the cranial T12 vertebra to the caudal T13 vertebra. The T2W hyperintensity in the spinal cord is most consistent with ischemic

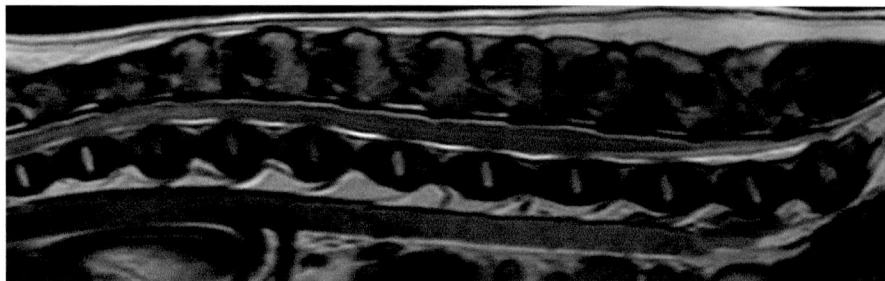

Fig. 5.8. T2W sagittal image of the lumbar spinal cord in Case 6. Note the intraparenchymal T2W hyperintensity over the 12th and 13th thoracic vertebrae. The lesion was not contrast-enhancing. (Image used with permission from Dr. Susan Arnold.)

myelopathy from a fibrocartilaginous embolism, or less likely contusion from an ANNPE. This intraparenchymal lesion is the most likely cause of the patient's clinical signs (Fig. 5.8).

Case conclusion

The dog's findings are consistent with FCEM. A dislodged piece of fibrocartilage, presumptively from a nearby intervertebral disc, enters a blood vessel that supplies the spinal cord, causing focal ischemia. FCEM most commonly affects large-breed, active dogs, but is also seen in higher frequency in Miniature Schnauzers (Hawthorne *et al.*, 2001). FCEM classically causes an activity-associated, peracute, nonprogressive myelopathy. The dog may vocalize at the onset but will not display evidence of pain or discomfort on vertebral column palpation. It is common for the signs to be moderately to markedly worse on one side than the other. No medical or surgical intervention is known to result in rapid resolution of clinical signs, therefore supportive care is often recommended. This dog's clinical signs gradually returned to normal with physical rehabilitation and supportive care including sling support and bladder function monitoring at home.

Case 7

Patient signalment

An 11-year-old neutered male domestic short-haired cat.

History

The cat was presented for a 2-month history of progressive difficulty using his pelvic limbs. The cat was started on prednisolone (2 mg PO q24h) about

7 weeks prior to presentation which initially led to substantial improvement for the first 6 weeks of treatment. However, the cat's neurologic dysfunction subsequently worsened, and he began urinating only once every 24 h. He was up to date on his vaccinations. He was an indoor-only cat with no travel history and ate a commercial cat food.

Physical examination

T: 38.7°C/101.6°F   P: 160 beats/min   R: 28 breaths/min

- **EENT:** Normal; no palpable thyroid slip.
- **Lymph nodes:** Soft, small, symmetrical.
- **Oropharyngeal:** Normal.
- **Integument:** Normal.
- **Musculoskeletal:** Moderate generalized muscle atrophy of both pelvic limbs.
- **Abdominal palpation:** Extremely distended, firm bladder on palpation. Abdominal splinting occurred with any degree of abdominal palpation.
- **Urogenital:** When penis was extruded, it was observed to be purple, with gritty, brown discharge dripping out of it. A small amount of blood was observed when the penis was wiped with a piece of gauze.
- **Respiratory:** Normal.
- **Cardiac:** Grade II/VI left apical systolic murmur. Strong, synchronous femoral pulses in both pelvic limbs, and limbs felt warm to the touch.

Neurologic examination

- **Mentation:** BAR.
- **Cranial nerve exam:** Normal.
- **Spinal reflexes:** Normal reflexes. Cutaneous trunci reflex not observed bilaterally. Normal perianal reflex and anal tone.
- **Postural reactions:** Normal in thoracic limbs. Absent paw replacement and hopping in both pelvic limbs.
- **Gait assessment:** Nonambulatory with severe paraparesis.
- **Spinal palpation:** No overt pain on palpation.
- **Cervical range of motion:** Normal.
- **Other:** Decreased muscle mass bilaterally in epaxial muscles. Increased tone appreciated in both pelvic limbs. No motor function observed in the tail. Nociception positive in the tail.

Neuroanatomic lesion localization practice sheet

Use this space below to work through NALL for Case 7. When you have finished, turn to the answer section on the following page to check your answers.

Abnormality	Possible NALL	Possible NALL	Possible NALL	Possible NALL	Possible NALL	Possible NALL

Discussion on neuroanatomic lesion localization

Abnormality	Possible NALL	Possible NALL	Possible NALL	Possible NALL	Possible NALL	Possible NALL	Possible NALL	Possible NALL
Nonambulatory paraparesis	Forebrain/ prosencephalon	Brainstem	C1–C5 myelopathy	C6–T2 myelopathy	T3–L3 myelopathy	L4–S3 myelopathy/ radiculopathy	Peripheral neuropathy	Myopathy
Absent pelvic limb postural reactions	Forebrain/ prosencephalon	Brainstem	C1–C5 myelopathy	C6–T2 myelopathy	T3–L3 myelopathy	L4–S3 myelopathy/ radiculopathy	Peripheral neuropathy	
Absent motor function in tail	Forebrain/ prosencephalon	Brainstem	C1–C5 myelopathy	C6–T2 myelopathy	T3–L3 myelopathy	T3–L3 myelopathy	S1–S3	Coccygeal muscles

Neuroanatomic lesion localization, Case 7: T3–L3 myelopathy

Begin by identifying a lack of signs of intracranial disease including seizures, cranial nerve deficits, mentation changes, or cerebellar gait abnormalities. The lesion is not intracranial in this cat. Thoracic limb abnormalities were not detected, therefore C1–C5 and C6–T2 spinal cord segments can be eliminated as possible NALL. This leaves a possible lesion localization of a T3–L3 or L4–S3 myelopathy or neuromuscular abnormalities affecting only the pelvic limb nerves or muscles. Normal reflexes were identified, therefore neuromuscular disease is unlikely. Although a myopathy may cause paraparesis with normal reflexes, that was ruled out due to identification of paw replacement deficits in the pelvic limbs. Furthermore, pets with lesions in the PNS typically have decreased to absent muscle tone. Finally, non-neurologic causes such as a distal aortic thromboembolism ("saddle thrombus") leading to loss of blood supply to the pelvic limb nerves and muscles is ruled out due to the presence of spinal reflexes and lack of pain on palpation. Additionally, this patient had strong femoral pulses and warm distal extremities.

A T3–L3 or L4–S3 myelopathy may now be considered. A lesion in the L4–S3 region of the spinal cord would result in loss of pelvic limb reflexes and loss of pelvic limb tone. Neither of these abnormalities was observed in this cat. Therefore, a T3–L3 myelopathy is the only possible lesion localization to explain the pelvic limb dysfunction in this case. In a T3–L3 myelopathy, the paraparesis results from loss of descending motor projections. These pathways consist of the UMNs that control voluntary activity. These UMNs synapse with the LMNs in the spinal cord and are generally inhibitory to the LMNs. In effect, a lesion affecting the UMNs results in UMN paresis, which is characterized by spastic paresis or paralysis and increased muscle tone. Spinal reflexes may become hyperreflexive. Importantly, patients with T3–L3 myelopathies will not have decreased pelvic limb spinal reflexes.

The lack of a cutaneous trunci reflex is most likely a reflection of a normal species variant rather than a true deficit. The cutaneous trunci reflex is unreliable in cats (Paushter *et al.*, 2020). Furthermore, the infrequent urination is due to his T3–L3 myelopathy. Not only is the cat unable to access his litterbox, but his T3–L3 myelopathy has also resulted in disruption of UMN innervation of his bladder and external urethral sphincter. This results in a spastic paresis/paralysis of the external urethral sphincter and detrusor muscles. The bladder is firm and overflow incontinence develops when the pressure of urine in the bladder exceeds the tone of the external urethral sphincter (Granger *et al.*, 2020).

Differential diagnoses

Slowly progressive, prednisone-responsive, T3–L3 myelopathy in a cat may be secondary to intervertebral disc herniation, neoplasia, or meningomyelitis.

Diagnostic testing and results

- **CBC:** Normal.
- **Serum biochemistry panel:** Normal.
- **ECG:** Left ventricular wall thickening with normal left atrial size, dynamic right ventricular outflow tract obstruction, systolic anterior motion of the mitral valve.
- **Thoracolumbar MRI:** Arising off the T13 dorsal lamina, a mass is present, resulting in severe extradural spinal cord compression. This mass most likely represents a malignant neoplasm, such as osteosarcoma, or alternatively other primary bone neoplasms or round cell neoplasia. Sternal lymphadenopathy is also present and is concerning for metastatic or multicentric neoplasia (Fig. 5.9).

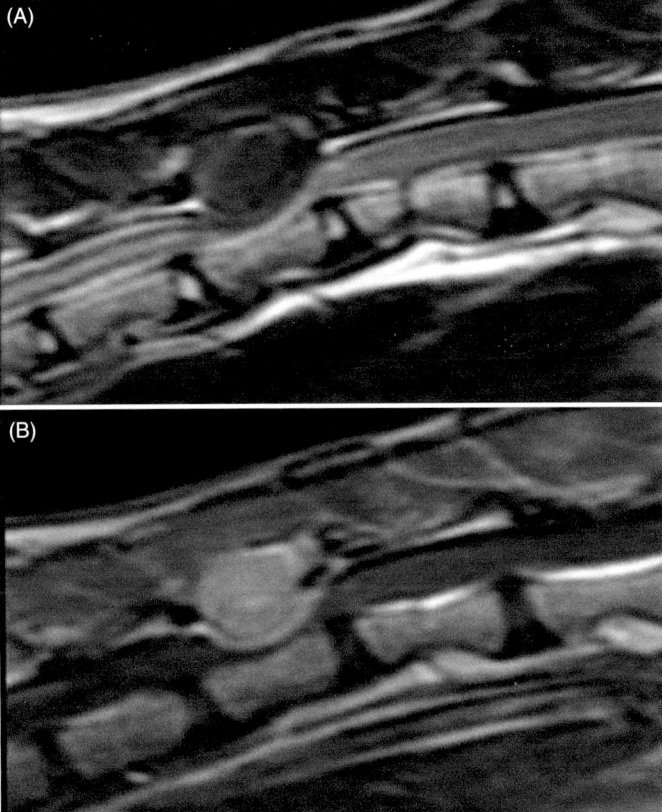

Fig. 5.9. T2W sagittal image (A) and T1W post-contrast image (B) of the thoracic spinal cord in Case 7. Image is hypointense to spinal cord on T2W imaging, and uniformly contrast-enhancing post contrast. (Images used with permission from Dr. Susan Arnold.)

Case conclusion

Surgical resection with possible radiation therapy and chemotherapy to fol-
low, continued palliative care, or euthanasia were discussed with the owner.
The cat's owner elected to surgically remove the mass. Surgical resection was
successful, and the mass was histopathologically confirmed to be an osteosarcoma. Osteosarcoma is reported to be the second most common tumor affecting the spinal cord noted on postmortem examination in cats (Marioni-Henry,
2010). Two weeks after surgery, the cat was ambulatory, comfortable, and voluntarily urinating. His owner acknowledged the likely metastasis given the sternal lymphadenopathy but elected not to proceed with further care. Follow-up 3
months later confirmed that he remained ambulatory and was able to run and
jump without detectable discomfort.

Case 8

Patient signalment

A 4-year-old male intact Abyssinian dog.

History

The dog was presented for a history of back pain that had been noted intermittently since adoption. The dog was born in Africa and moved to the USA 2
years prior to presentation. In cold weather, the dog demonstrated reluctance
to climb on or off furniture in the home but was otherwise an active dog. He
did not have a history of trauma.

Physical examination

T: 39.3°C/102.8°F   P: 120 beats/min   R: panting

- **EENT:** Anxious, therefore a limited oral and facial examination was performed.
- **Lymph nodes:** No abnormalities detected.
- **Oropharyngeal:** Did not evaluate.
- **Integument:** No ectoparasites, otherwise normal examination.
- **Musculoskeletal:** No abnormalities noted.
- **Abdominal palpation:** No abnormalities detected.
- **Urogenital:** No abnormalities on external genitalia.
- **Respiratory:** Normal.
- **Cardiac:** No arrythmia or murmur noted.

Neurologic examination

- **Mentation:** BAR.
- **Cranial nerve exam:** Normal.
- **Spinal reflexes:** Normal reflexes; normal cutaneous trunci and perineal reflexes.
- **Postural reactions:** Normal in thoracic limbs; absent paw replacement in both pelvic limbs.
- **Gait assessment:** Ambulatory with a kyphotic posture and mild paraparesis.
- **Spinal palpation:** Marked multifocal spinal hyperpathia at upper thoracic, mid-thoracic, and lumbosacral regions.
- **Cervical range of motion:** Normal.
- **Other:** None.

Neuroanatomic lesion localization practice sheet

Use this space below to work through NALL for Case 8. When you have finished, turn to the answer section on the following page to check your answers.

Abnormality	Possible NALL	Possible NALL	Possible NALL	Possible NALL	Possible NALL	Possible NALL

Discussion on neuroanatomic lesion localization

Abnormality	Possible NALL	Possible NALL	Possible NALL	Possible NALL	Possible NALL	Possible NALL	Possible NALL	Possible NALL
Nonambulatory paraparesis	Forebrain/ prosencephalon	Brainstem	C1–C5 myelopathy	C6–T2 myelopathy	T3–L3 myelopathy	L4–S3 myelopathy/ radiculopathy	Peripheral neuropathy	Myopathy
Absent pelvic limb postural reactions	Forebrain/ prosencephalon	Brainstem	C1–C5 myelopathy	C6–T2 myelopathy	T3–L3 myelopathy	L4–S3 myelopathy/ radiculopathy	Peripheral neuropathy	
Absent motor function in tail	Forebrain/ prosencephalon	Brainstem	C1–C5 myelopathy	C6–T2 myelopathy	T3–L3 myelopathy	T3–L3 myelopathy	S1–S3	Coccygeal muscles

Neuroanatomic lesion localization, Case 8: T3–L3 myelopathy

Begin by identifying a lack of signs of intracranial disease including seizures, cranial nerve deficits, mentation changes, or cerebellar gait abnormalities. The lesion is not intracranial in this dog. Thoracic limb abnormalities were not detected, therefore C1–C5 and C6–T2 spinal cord segments can be eliminated as possible NALL. This leaves a possible lesion localization of a T3–L3 or L4–S3 myelopathy or neuromuscular abnormalities affecting only the pelvic limb nerves or muscles. Normal reflexes were identified, therefore neuromuscular disease is unlikely, as is an L4–S3 myelopathy.

A T3–L3 myelopathy may now be considered. Multifocal spinal pain within this region could suggest a multifocal lesion within the T3–L3 spinal cord region, or focal pain with referred pain to other spinal locations.

Differential diagnoses

Minimally progressive spinal pain with evidence of a T3–L3 myelopathy is suggestive of intervertebral disc herniation (type II), neoplasia, or discospondlyitis. Meningomyelitis was considered; however the prolonged clinical history of several years makes this differential diagnosis unlikely.

Diagnostic testing and results

- **CBC:** Normal.
- **Serum biochemistry panel:** Normal.
- **Thoracolumbar radiographs:** Lysis was noted at the end plates of L3–L4 and at the articular processes of T13–L1 and L4–L5. This finding is most consistent with osteomyelitis with discospondylitis; however osseous neoplasia could not be ruled out (Kewin *et al.*, 1992) (Fig. 5.10).
- ***B. canis* rapid slide agglutination test:** Positive.
- ***B canis* 2-mercaptoethanol tube agglutination test:** Positive.

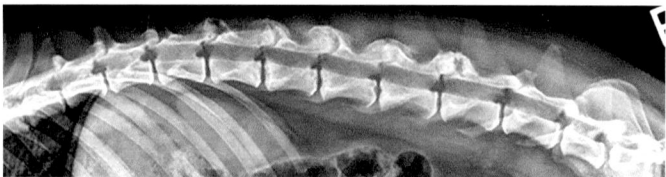

Fig. 5.10. Lateral radiograph of the thoracolumbar region of Case 8. Lysis is evident at the L3–L4 end plates and articular processes of T13–L1 and L4–L5.

Case conclusion

This dog was diagnosed with suspected osteomyelitis and discospondylitis of multiple vertebrae in the thoracolumbar region secondary to *Brucella canis* infection. *B. canis* is a gram-negative coccobacillus rarely diagnosed in the USA but may be found more commonly in other countries. Due to the risk of zoonotic transmission, humane euthanasia was recommended (Cosford, 2018). The family elected to pursue treatment; therefore the dog was treated with minocycline and enrofloxacin, and quarantine away from dogs and humans was recommended. Appropriate personal protective gear was worn when handling the dog, or any laboratory samples, to avoid human transmission, and minimal hospitalization was recommended when evaluating the dog (Ruoff *et al.*, 2018).

References

Cosford, K.L. (2018) *Brucella canis*: an update on research and clinical management. *Canadian Veterinary Journal* 59(1), 74–81. Available at: https://www.ncbi.nlm.nih.gov/pmc/articles/PMC5731389/pdf/cvj_01_74.pdf (accessed 9 June 2022).

De Decker, S., da Costa, R.C., Volk, H.A. and Van Ham, L.M.L. (2012) Current insights and controversies in the pathogenesis and diagnosis of disc-associated cervical spondylomyelopathy in dogs. *Veterinary Record* 171(21), 531–537. doi: 10.1136/vr.e7952.

de Lahunta, A. and Glass, E. (2009) *Veterinary Neuroanatomy and Clinical Neurology*, 3rd edn. Saunders Elsevier, St. Louis, Missouri.

Granger, N., Olby, N.J. and Nout-Lomas, Y.S. (2020) Bladder and bowel management in dogs with spinal cord injury. *Frontiers in Veterinary Science* 7, 583342. doi: 10.3389/fvets.2020.583342.

Havig, M.E., Cornell, K.K., Hawthorne, J.C., McDonnell, J.J. and Selcer, B.A. (2005) Evaluation of nonsurgical treatment of atlantoaxial subluxation in dogs: 19 cases (1992–2001). *Journal of the American Veterinary Medical Association* 227(2), 257–262.

Hawthorne, J.C., Wallace, L.J., Fenner, W.R. and Waters, D.J. (2001) Fibrocartilaginous embolic myelopathy in miniature schnauzers. *Journal of the American Animal Hospital Association* 37(4), 374–383. doi: 10.5326/15473317-37-4-374.

Kewin, S., Lewis, D. and Hribernik, T. (1992) Diskospondylitis associated with *Brucella canis* infection in dogs: 14 cases (1980–1991). *Journal of the American Veterinary Medical Association* 201(8), 1253–1257.

Marioni-Henry, K. (2010) Feline spinal cord diseases. *Veterinary Clinics of North America: Small Animal Practice* 40(5), 1011–1028. doi: 10.1016/j.cvsm.2010.05.005.

Pancotto, T.E., Rossmeisl, J.H. Jr, Zimmerman, K., Robertson, J.L. and Were, S.R. (2013) Intramedullary spinal cord neoplasia in 53 dogs (1990–2010): distribution, clinicopathologic characteristics, and clinical behavior. *Journal of Veterinary Internal Medicine* 27(6), 1500–1508. doi: 10.1111/jvim.12182.

Paushter, A.M., Hague, D.W., Foss, K.D. and Sander, W.E. (2020) Assessment of the cutaneous trunci muscle reflex in neurologically abnormal cats. *Journal of Feline Medicine and Surgery* 22(12), 1200–1205. doi: 10.1177/1098612X20917810.

Rodiño-Tilve, V., Guevar, J., Hammond, G. and Penderis, J. (2017) Incomplete ossification of the atlas in a dog: surgical stabilisation using a SOP plate. *Journal of Small Animal Practice* 58(5), 301. doi: 10.1111/jsap.12664.

Ruoff, C.M., Kerwin, S.C. and Taylor, A.R. (2018) Diagnostic imaging of discospondylitis. *Veterinary Clinics of North America: Small Animal Practice* 48(1), 85–94. doi: 10.1016/j. cvsm.2017.08.007.

Sharp, N. and Wheeler, S.J. (2004) *Small Animal Spinal Disorders*, 2nd edn. Elsevier Mosby, St. Louis, Missouri.

Slanina, M.C. (2016) Atlantoaxial instability. *Veterinary Clinics of North America: Small Animal Practice* 46(2), 265–275. doi: 10.1016/j.cvsm.2015.10.005.

Warren-Smith, C., Kneissl, S., Benigni, L., Kenny, P.J. and Lamb, C.R. (2009) Incomplete ossification of the atlas in dogs with cervical signs. *Veterinary Radiology & Ultrasound* 50(6), 635–638. doi: 10.1111/j.1740-8261.2009.01595.x.

6   Neuromuscular Disease

Heidi Barnes Heller[1]*, Kari Foss[2] and Sam Long[3]

[1]Barnes Veterinary Specialty Services, Madison, Wisconsin, USA;
[2]University of Illinois, Urbana, Illinois, USA; [3]Veterinary Referral Hospital,
Dandenong, Victoria, Australia

Unless otherwise noted, all images and videos are owned by the lead author.

Case 1

Patient signalment

A 5-year-old castrated male German Shepherd dog.

History

The patient presented for progressive tetraparesis of 5 days' duration. Five days prior to presentation the dog was noted to have several cuts on his nose when the owners let him back inside. The following day, the dog appeared to be walking slower with a limp on the right pelvic limb. Carprofen (dose unknown) was prescribed without clinical improvement. Thoracic limb stumbling was noted 3 days later with subsequent progression to an inability to walk on all four limbs over the next 24 h.

The patient has a history of a right cranial crucial ligament rupture with surgical correction and secondary osteoarthritis 4 years prior to this evaluation. Additionally, the dog lives on a rural property with four other dogs.

*Email: barnes@barnesveterinaryservices.com

© CAB International 2022. *Small Animal Neuroanatomic Lesion Localization Practice Book*
(ed. H. Barnes Heller)
DOI: 10.1079/9781789247947.0006

Physical examination

T: 38.1°C/100.6°F   P: 90 beats/min   R: 50/min

- **EENT:** Clear corneas, no abnormalities noted.
- **Lymph nodes:** Normal, no peripheral lymphadenopathy noted.
- **Oropharyngeal:** Pink mucous membranes, normal CRT, no masses seen.
- **Integument:** Euhydrated; small, superficial, healing laceration on nose.
- **Musculoskeletal:** Discomfort on hyperextension of hips and slightly effusive right stifle.
- **Abdominal palpation:** Normal, soft, nonpainful, no masses or organomegaly noted.
- **Urogenital:** Grossly normal.
- **Respiratory:** No nasal discharge, no tracheal sensitivity, lungs clear.
- **Cardiac:** No murmur or arrhythmia.

Neurologic examination

- **Mentation:** BAR.
- **Cranial nerve exam:** No abnormalities noted.
- **Spinal reflexes:** Severely decreased to absent withdrawal reflexes in all four limbs; decreased patellar reflexes bilaterally. Decreased muscle tone in all four limbs.
- **Postural reactions:** Hopping intact in all four limbs when given adequate support; placing delayed in all four limbs.
- **Gait assessment:** Nonambulatory tetraparesis with minimal motor function in the pelvic limbs and moderate motor function in the thoracic limbs. Lateralization to one side or the other was not present (Video 6.1).
- **Spinal palpation:** No paraspinal pain elicited on palpation.
- **Cervical range of motion:** Normal.
- **Other:** Mild, generalized muscle atrophy noted, most prominent over limbs.

Video 6.1. Video of Case 1 showing a nonambulatory tetraparesis with minimal motor function in the pelvic limbs and moderate motor function in the thoracic limbs. Lateralization was not present. (Video used with permission from Dr. Kari Foss.) (https://vimeo.com/696921886; video.cabi.org/SMUAI)

Neuroanatomic lesion localization practice sheet

Use this space below to work through NALL for Case 1. When you have finished, turn to the answer section on the following page to check your answers.

Abnormality	Possible NALL	Possible NALL	Possible NALL	Possible NALL	Possible NALL	Possible NALL

Discussion on neuroanatomic lesion localization

Abnormality	Possible NALL	Possible NALL	Possible NALL	Possible NALL	Possible NALL	Possible NALL
Tetraparesis	Forebrain/ prosencephalon	Brainstem	C1–C5 myelopathy	C6–T2 myelopathy	Peripheral neuropathy	Neuromuscular junction
Absent spinal reflexes				C6–T2 AND L4–S3	Peripheral neuropathy	Neuromuscular junction
Delayed placing responses, all four limbs	Forebrain/ prosencephalon	Brainstem	C1–C5 myelopathy	C6–T2 myelopathy	Peripheral neuropathy	Neuromuscular junction

Neuroanatomic lesion localization, Case 1: Neuromuscular

The NALL is neuromuscular. Paresis, without evidence of ataxia, suggests a neuromuscular cause rather than a spinal cause. In the neuromuscular system there are three localizations commonly used: peripheral neuropathy, neuromuscular junction, and myopathy. Patients with a peripheral neuropathy often demonstrate reduced reflexes; those with neuromuscular junction disease often have absent reflexes; and those with myopathies are expected to have normal reflexes despite often severe weakness. Based on the severely reduced reflexes in all four limbs, neuromuscular junction is the most likely site for the neuromuscular signs in this dog, however a severe peripheral neuropathy cannot be excluded.

Differential diagnoses

Given the patient's history and unspecified injury (scratches on nose), the most likely differential diagnosis is canine APN (coonhound paralysis). Other differential diagnoses include fulminant myasthenia gravis, tick paralysis, coral snake envenomation, and less likely botulism (Cuddon, 2002).

Diagnostic testing and results

- **CBC:** No clinically significant abnormalities.
- **Chemistry panel:** CPK = 93 U/l (normal, 26–791 U/l), all remaining results within normal parameters.
- **Thoracic radiographs:** No evidence of metastatic disease or megaesophagus.
- **AChR antibody titer:** 0.13 nmol/l (normal serum titer, < 0.6 nmol/l).

Case conclusion

The final diagnosis for this case was canine APN (coonhound paralysis) (Halstead et al., 2022). The patient was hospitalized for supportive care and twice-daily inpatient physical therapy was performed. Continued progression was noted during the first several days of hospitalization to include absent withdrawal reflexes in all limbs, absent patellar reflexes bilaterally, and tetraplegia. Over the course of 2 weeks supportive care and rehabilitation therapy were continued, and slow improvement was noted with return of spinal reflexes (still markedly decreased) and the presence of minimal motor function. The patient was discharged in a state of nonambulatory tetraparesis along with instructions for continued supportive care and rehabilitation at home.

Two months later the patient was ambulatory with mild tetraparesis. Withdrawal reflexes and patellar reflexes were slightly decreased in all limbs. Subsequently the patient was lost to follow-up.

Case 2

Patient signalment

A 3-year-old spayed female Boxer dog.

History

The patient presented with a 6-month history of progressive muscle tremors, generalized weakness, and weight loss. Six months prior to evaluation, the patient developed difficulty walking in her pelvic limbs and a decreased appetite. Oral prednisone (dose unknown) was prescribed by the local veterinarian. Signs significantly improved on prednisone; therefore she was tapered off the medication after approximately 3 weeks. Upon discontinuation of the steroids, the clinical signs of pelvic limb weakness began to return. One month prior to presentation the patient became progressively weaker becoming poorly ambulatory. Despite continuing to eat and drink normally, the patient also lost a significant amount of weight. An AChR antibody titer was negative.

Physical examination

T: 38.3°C/101.0°F   P: 101 beats/min   R: 18 breaths/min

- **EENT:** Clear corneas, no abnormalities noted.
- **Lymph nodes:** Normal, no peripheral lymphadenopathy noted.
- **Oropharyngeal:** Pink mucous membranes, normal CRT, no masses seen.
- **Integument:** No abnormalities detected.
- **Musculoskeletal:** Moderate generalized muscle atrophy.
- **Abdominal palpation:** Normal, soft, nonpainful, no masses or organomegaly noted.
- **Urogenital:** Grossly normal.
- **Respiratory:** No nasal discharge, no tracheal sensitivity, lungs clear.
- **Cardiac:** No murmur or arrhythmia.

Neurologic examination

- **Mentation:** BAR.
- **Cranial nerve exam:** No abnormalities noted.
- **Spinal reflexes:** Withdrawal reflexes were decreased in all four limbs. Markedly decreased to absent patellar reflexes bilaterally (Video 6.2).
- **Postural reactions:** Normal placing and hopping in all four limbs.
- **Gait assessment:** Ambulatory tetraparesis with short-stride gait in all four limbs. The patient is only able to support her body weight for about 30–40 s before lowering to sternal recumbency. No ataxia was noted.

- **Spinal palpation:** No paraspinal pain elicited on palpation.
- **Cervical range of motion:** Normal.
- **Other:** Generalized tremoring in all limbs when supporting body weight.

Video 6.2. Video of Case 2 showing ambulatory tetraparesis with short-stride gait in all four limbs. (Video used with permission from Dr. Kari Foss.) (https://vimeo.com/696940717; video.cabi.org/QZCIQ)

Neuroanatomic lesion localization practice sheet

Use this space below to work through NALL for Case 2. When you have finished, turn to the answer section on the following page to check your answers.

Abnormality	Possible NALL	Possible NALL	Possible NALL	Possible NALL	Possible NALL	Possible NALL

Discussion on neuroanatomic lesion localization

Abnormality	Possible NALL	Possible NALL	Possible NALL	Possible NALL	Possible NALL	Possible NALL	Possible NALL
Tetraparesis	Forebrain/ prosencephalon	Brainstem	C1–C5 myelopathy	C6–T2 myelopathy	Peripheral neuropathy	Neuromuscular junction
Delayed spinal reflexes				C6–T2 AND L4–S3	Peripheral neuropathy	Neuromuscular junction
Tremors when standing	Myopathy	Non-neurologic causes				

Neuroanatomic lesion localization, Case 2: Neuromuscular

The NALL is neuromuscular. Tetraparesis without ataxia suggests that the CNS is not affected. Therefore, a neuromuscular lesion localization should be considered. Normal to reduced reflexes would be consistent with a peripheral neuropathy, early neuromuscular disease, or myopathy in which severe muscle atrophy results in reduced magnitude of the reflexes. Without additional testing, it is difficult to determine which neuroanatomic neuromuscular localization is causing the clinical signs in this case.

Differential diagnoses

Differential diagnoses including peripheral neuropathic causes such as protozoal diseases (*Toxoplasma gondii* and *Neospora caninum*), fungal neuropathy, immune-mediated polyneuritis, and paraneoplastic peripheral neuropathy were considered. Causes of neuromuscular junction disease such as myasthenia gravis or early polyradiculoneuritis may also be considered. Finally, causes of myopathy such as immune-mediated polymyositis, infectious myositis (protozoal most common), and paraneoplastic myositis were considered.

Diagnostic testing and results

- **Serum CK:** Markedly elevated (6281 U/l; reference range, 26–310 U/l).
- *Toxoplasma* **IgG titer/IgM screen:** Negative IgM, negative IgG.
- **Tick panel PCR:** Negative for *Anaplasma, Babesia, Bartonella, Ehrlichia,* and *Rickettsia.*
- **Abdominal ultrasound:** Mild gallbladder sludge—otherwise unremarkable.
- **EMG:** Marked abnormal spontaneous muscle activity was noted in multiple muscles in the pelvic and thoracic limbs, as well as the epaxial musculature, and muscles of mastication (temporalis and masseter). These findings were consistent with either muscle disease or denervation (nerve disorder) (Video 6.3).
- **Nerve and muscle biopsies:** Unfixed and fixed biopsies were submitted from the cranial tibial and extensor carpi radialis muscles. Except for mild variability in myofiber size and minimal to mild mononuclear cell infiltration, no specific abnormalities were identified in the muscle and nerve biopsies. Given the minimal to mild cellular infiltrations and high CK activity, an inflammatory myopathy/myositis is most likely (Evans *et al.,* 2004). Inflammatory myopathies can have a patchy distribution and areas of more marked cellular infiltration may be present in other muscle groups. If infectious causes of myositis can be ruled out (*Toxoplasma, Neospora,* or tick-related diseases), an immune-mediated (polymyositis) or paraneoplastic syndrome should be considered. No abnormalities were found in the biopsy from the peroneal nerve.

Video 6.3. Needle EMG of Case 2. Findings include marked spontaneous activity including positive sharp waves and fibrillation potentials. Findings were noted in pelvic and thoracic limbs, along with the epaxial muscles and the muscles of mastication. (Video used with permission from Dr. Keri Foss.) (https://vimeo.com/696940898; video.cabi.org/MEQHA)

Case conclusion

The patient was diagnosed with polymyositis with a suspected immune-mediated cause due to the lack of evidence of infectious disease (Hankel *et al.*, 2006). Prednisone (2 mg/kg PO q24h) and gabapentin (10 mg/kg PO q8h) were prescribed, and clinical improvement was noted within 72 h after starting medications. Clinical signs worsened 4 days later, on the same dose of prednisone but after discontinuing gabapentin. The owners elected humane euthanasia.

Case 3

Patient signalment

A 6-year-old castrated male Akita.

History

The dog was presented for further work-up of hyporexia, weakness, lethargy, and difficulty prehending food. CBC, serum chemistry, pancreatic lipase, resting cortisol, heartworm test, and a canine SNAP 4Dx Plus panel were performed by the primary veterinarian and were normal. The dog was presented to the emergency room for continued difficulty eating and found to have a persistent sinus tachycardia based on ECG, which also showed a small left ventricle and an overall decreased size to the cardiac silhouette. These findings along with the sinus were suggestive of hypovolemia. The patient was admitted and received IV fluid therapy. Additional testing prior to presentation also included an ACTH stimulation test and thoracic radiographs, which were both normal. A urine *Blastomyces* antigen test was also negative.

On presentation to the neurology and neurosurgery service a week later, the patient was reported to be doing better, although he still had mild dysphagia when eating and drinking. The patient had also been having some loose stools. Medication on presentation included metronidazole (20 mg/kg PO q12h), amoxicillin/clavulanic acid (18 mg/kg PO q12h), carprofen (4 mg/kg PO q24h), omeprazole (0.5 mg/kg PO q12h), and Proviable DC (1 capsule PO q24h).

Physical examination

T: 39.9°C/103.8 °F   P: 104 beats/min   R: panting

- **EENT:** Clear corneas, no abnormalities noted.
- **Lymph nodes:** Normal, no peripheral lymphadenopathy noted.
- **Oropharyngeal:** Pink mucous membranes, normal CRT, no masses seen.
- **Integument:** Euhydrated, coat healthy.
- **Musculoskeletal:** Bilateral masseter and temporalis muscle atrophy. Ambulatory all four limbs.
- **Abdominal palpation:** Normal, soft, nonpainful, no masses or organomegaly noted.
- **Urogenital:** Grossly normal.
- **Respiratory:** No nasal discharge, no tracheal sensitivity, lungs clear.
- **Cardiac:** No murmur or arrhythmia. Strong synchronous pulses.

Neurologic examination

- **Mentation:** BAR.
- **Cranial nerve exam:** Significant atrophy of the temporalis and masseter muscles; slightly decreased gag reflex.
- **Spinal reflexes:** Decreased withdrawal reflexes in all four limbs. Decreased patellar reflexes bilaterally.
- **Postural reactions:** Placing and hopping intact in all four limbs.
- **Gait assessment:** Mild tetraparesis (worsens with activity); no ataxia or lameness noted.
- **Spinal palpation:** No paraspinal pain elicited on palpation.
- **Cervical range of motion:** Normal.
- **Other:** Mild, generalized muscle atrophy noted, most prominent over limbs.

Neuroanatomic lesion localization practice sheet

Use this space below to work through NALL for Case 3. When you have finished, turn to the answer section on the following page to check your answers.

Abnormality	Possible NALL	Possible NALL	Possible NALL	Possible NALL	Possible NALL	Possible NALL

Discussion on neuroanatomic lesion localization

Abnormality	Possible NALL	Possible NALL	Possible NALL	Possible NALL	Possible NALL	Possible NALL	Possible NALL
Tetraparesis	Forebrain/ prosencephalon	Brainstem	C1–C5 myelopathy	C6–T2 myelopathy	Peripheral neuropathy	Neuromuscular junction
Temporalis and masseter atrophy	Myopathy	Bilateral trigeminal neuropathy					
Reduced gag reflex	CN IX	Cranial nerve 10	Medulla oblongata				
Reduced withdrawal reflexes all limbs	C6–T2 and L6–S3 myelopathy	Peripheral neuropathy	Neuromuscular junction	Severe myopathy with severe muscle atrophy			
Reduced patellar reflexes bilaterally	L4–L6 myelopathy	Femoral neuropathy	Neuromuscular junction				

Neuroanatomic lesion localization, Case 3: Neuromuscular

The dog in this case had evidence of tetraparesis, suggesting this could be a spinal lesion, neuromuscular lesion, or less likely an intracranial cause. It is important to remember that dogs and cats with spinal cord disease will almost always have a loss of proprioceptive testing before paresis, and certainly before profound paresis. By identifying a lack of ataxia in this dog, the NALL is automatically narrowed to the neuromuscular system. Within the neuromuscular system, the NALL can be further narrowed to a peripheral neuropathy, neuromuscular junctionopathy, or a myopathy. Animals with a peripheral neuropathy are expected to have reduced to absent reflexes in multiple locations; animals with neuromuscular junction disease are expected to have a complete loss of reflexes; and animals with a myopathy are expected to have normal reflexes—however, with severe muscle atrophy or disease, reduced reflexes may sometimes be noted. In this case, the reduced reflexes with an ambulatory dog lead the evaluator to suspect a peripheral neuropathy.

Differential diagnoses

Differential diagnoses including peripheral neuropathic causes such as protozoal diseases (*T. gondii* and *N. caninum*), fungal neuropathy, immune-mediated polyneuritis (including demyelinating polyneuropathy or denervating degeneration), and paraneoplastic peripheral neuropathy were considered. Finally, causes of myopathy such as metabolic causes (hyperadrenocorticism, hypothyroidism), polymyositis (immune mediated), infectious myositis, fulminant myasthenia gravis, and paraneoplastic myositis were considered.

Diagnostic testing and results

- **CBC:** Mild neutrophilia with slight toxic changes.
- **Chemistry panel:** Slight hypoalbuminemia, CK = 335 U/l (reference range, 10–200 U/l), AST = 70 U/l (reference range, 16–55 U/l).
- **Urine *Blastomyces* antigen:** Negative.
- **Urinalysis (while receiving IV fluids):** USG = 1.015, pH = 8, WBC = 15 cells/hpf.
- **Urine culture:** No growth.
- **ACTH stimulation:** Normal.
- **Thoracic radiographs:** No evidence of pleural effusion.
- **2M antibody test (masticatory muscle myositis):** Negative.
- **Thyroid:** Normal.
- **Biopsy of cranial tibial muscle:** Small intramuscular nerve branches were normal in appearance. Moderately excessive intramyofiber lipid droplets present within most type I fibers. No inflammation, necrosis, fibrosis, fiber loss, organisms, or other specific cytoarchitectural abnormalities were observed.

- **Biopsy of peroneal nerve:** The density and distribution of all calibers of nerve fibers were subjectively appropriate. No axonal degeneration, demyelination, or abnormalities of supporting structures were found.
- **Plasma amino acid panel:** Markedly elevated carnitine.
- **Urine organic acid panel:** Lactic acidosis with secondary elevation of 2-oxoisovaleric and 2-oxo-3-methylavleric. Normal 2-hydroxyisovaleric, 2-hydroxy-3-methylvaleric, and 2-oxoisocaproic. Elevation of 3-hydroxy-butyric with secondary elevations of acetoacetic and 3-hydroxyisobutyric. May be secondary to impending or resolving ketosis.
- **Urine carnitine levels:** Increased total carnitine (389.2 mmol/l; reference range, 0–32 mmol/l); increased free carnitine (348.1 mmol/l; reference range, 0–15 mmol/l).
- **Muscle carnitine levels:** Low free carnitine (3.2 µmol/kg protein; reference range, 5–18 µmol/kg protein).

Case conclusion

This patient was ultimately diagnosed with a myopathy, suspected to be caused by a lipid storage defect. Although the reduced reflexes suggested a neuropathy, the severe malfunction of the muscle was responsible for the reduced reflexes (de Lahunta and Glass, 2009; Skerritt, 2018). He was provided supplementation of L-carnitine (50 mg/kg PO q12h) and coenzyme Q10 with riboflavin (100 mg/day). Signs completely resolved with supplementation. The dog continued to remain clinically improved for several years and was euthanized for reasons unrelated to his myopathy.

Case 4

Patient signalment

A 3-year-old female spayed Smithfield terrier located in Victoria, Australia.

History

The dog presented for a history of progressive weakness over the preceding 7 days. Signs began with a fall off the outside deck at home (approximately 15 cm/1 ft off the ground) after which she was noted to stumble occasionally on both fore limbs and developed a right hind limb lameness. This progressed steadily to nonambulatory tetraparesis. At the point of presentation, she was unable to stand but could prop herself up into sternal recumbency for short periods of time. She was also noted to have had a change in voice with a weak bark. No other significant health issues were noted. She lives on a rural property with access to chickens and is fed a commercial diet but has been known to scavenge (the local kookaburras are fed chicken hearts as treats). She was initially seen by another specialist practice then referred to the neurology service.

Physical examination

T: 38.6°C/101.5°F   P: 100 beats/min   R: panting

- **EENT:** Within normal limits.
- **Lymph nodes:** Within normal limits.
- **Oropharyngeal:** Mucous membranes pink, CRT < 2 s, otherwise unremarkable.
- **Integument:** Within normal limits.
- **Musculoskeletal:** Within normal limits.
- **Abdominal palpation:** Within normal limits
- **Urogenital:** Within normal limits.
- **Respiratory:** Normal thoracic auscultation, no evidence of dyspnea or stridor.
- **Cardiac:** Normal (synchronous) femoral pulses, no audible murmur.

Neurologic examination

- **Mentation:** BAR.
- **Cranial nerve exam:** No abnormalities detected; normal gag and tongue movement noted on oral exam.
- **Spinal reflexes:** Withdrawal reflex absent in all four limbs, patellar reflex significantly decreased in both hind limbs but present. Biceps, triceps, extensor carpi radialis, gastrocnemius, and cranial tibial reflexes were significantly reduced. Generalized reduction in muscle tone in all appendicular muscles.
- **Postural reactions:** With support she made reasonable attempts to correct all four limbs on paw position and would attempt to hop when hopping was performed. Hemistanding/hemiwalking was not possible, given her weakness, nor was hip sway. When wheelbarrowed she would attempt to take reasonable steps but with no weight-bearing ability.
- **Gait assessment:** Nonambulatory. When placed in a standing position with assistance, she would try to bear weight for a few seconds on her fore limbs before collapsing. When lying she would be able to support herself in sternal recumbency briefly before collapsing into lateral recumbency.
- **Spinal palpation:** Within normal limits.
- **Cervical range of motion:** Within normal limits.
- **Other:** None.

Neuroanatomic lesion localization practice sheet

Use this space below to work through NALL for Case 4. When you have finished, turn to the answer section on the following page to check your answers.

Abnormality	Possible NALL	Possible NALL	Possible NALL	Possible NALL	Possible NALL	Possible NALL

Discussion on neuroanatomic lesion localization

Abnormality	Possible NALL	Possible NALL	Possible NALL	Possible NALL	Possible NALL	Possible NALL
Tetraparesis	Forebrain/prosencephalon	Brainstem	C1–C5 myelopathy	C6–T2 myelopathy	Peripheral neuropathy	Neuromuscular junction
Hypotonia	Peripheral neuropathy	Neuromuscular junction	Myopathy			
Dysphonia	CN IX	CN X	Medulla oblongata			
Absent withdrawal reflexes all limbs	C6–T2 and L6–S3 myelopathy	Peripheral neuropathy	Neuromuscular junction	Severe myopathy with severe muscle atrophy		
Reduced patellar reflexes bilaterally	L4–L6 myelopathy	Femoral neuropathy	Neuromuscular junction			

Neuroanatomic lesion localization, Case 4: Neuromuscular

The most striking feature of the dog's neurologic examination was generalized weakness, but with relatively good preservation of proprioceptive function— she was aware of the position of her limbs but had a dramatically reduced ability to replace them unless assisted (an important reminder of the need to support patient body weight while performing proprioceptive function tests). In general, neuromuscular weakness as a clinical problem is an indication of a condition affecting either multiple nerves (neuropathy) or muscles (myopathy), or the neuromuscular junctions (neuromuscular junctionopathy). The significant reduction in motor tone and reflex strength were more indicative of either an LMN disorder or a myopathy. Facial weakness and dysphonia are relatively common features of several causes of neuromuscular weakness.

Differential diagnoses

The differential diagnosis list for cases presenting with neuromuscular weakness generally looks something like the following (the most common causes are listed—more unusual, breed-specific diseases omitted).

- Neuropathic causes:
    - Tick paralysis (geography-specific).
    - Snake envenomation (geography-specific).
    - Tetrodotoxin ingestion (geography-specific).
    - APN/coonhound paralysis.
    - Hypothyroid neuropathy.
    - Paraneoplastic neuropathy.
    - Diabetic neuropathy.
    - CRIDP.
    - Botulism.
- Myopathic causes:
    - Immune-mediated polymyositis.
    - Congenital myopathies (e.g., muscular dystrophy).
    - Necrotizing myopathy.
    - Toxin-induced myopathy (monensin).
- Neuromuscular junctionopathy:
    - Myasthenia gravis.

Diagnostic testing and results

- **CBC/Biochemistry panel:** (only abnormalities listed) AST = 187 IU/l (range, 17–84 IU/l); CK = 1362 IU/l (range, 73–522 IU/l).
- **T4/TSH:** Total T4 = 21 nmol/l (range, 13–47 nmol/l); TSH = 0.08 ng/ml (range, 0.1–0.45 ng/ml).
- **Cortisol:** 100 nmol/l (> 55 nmol/l excludes hypoadrenocorticism).

- **Urinalysis:** Unremarkable (with no growth on culture/sensitivity).
- **Thoracic radiographs:** Unremarkable.
- **Abdominal ultrasound:** Unremarkable.
- **EMG/Nerve conduction velocity:** Mild fibrillation potentials/positive sharp waves were found in multiple muscle groups (most pronounced in the gastrocnemius muscles) along with markedly delayed CMAPs. Repetitive nerve stimulation was within normal limits. These findings suggested a proximal neuropathy.
- **AChR antibody testing:** 0.10 nmol/l (normal, 0–0.60 nmol/l).

Case conclusion

Following diagnostic testing the dog was diagnosed with APN and was managed in hospital for the following 8 days before being discharged into the care of her owners (Halstead *et al.*, 2022). The elevated CK and AST levels were presumed to be the result of prolonged recumbency. In addition, 24 h of oral pyridostigmine (1 mg/kg q8h) were given but no significant improvement was noted and so this was discontinued. During hospitalization she was managed for urine scalding and kept on a soft bed and turned every 4 h to prevent the development of pressure sores. Passive range of motion and oral care were performed. Approximately 5 days post admission she was noted to be producing dark, foul-smelling urine which prompted cystocentesis and submission of urine for urinalysis, culture, and sensitivity. A moderate growth of *Enterococcus fecalis* was isolated that was sensitive to amoxicillin–clavulanic acid, which was instigated, and which resolved the urinary tract infection (secondary to prolonged recumbency). She remained nonambulatory for the duration of her hospital stay and for several weeks at home before regaining strength and the ability to walk and run normally. In our clinic we hospitalize patients for long enough post diagnosis to ensure no further deterioration is occurring (in particular, focusing on respiratory function to ensure ventilation is not required) and cannot overemphasize the importance of good nursing care in the treatment of these patients. Full recovery took approximately 12 weeks post admission for this dog.

Investigating these cases requires a methodical, step-by-step ruling out of all the possible differential diagnoses. The neurologic examination was most suspicious for a disorder affecting LMNs and predominately sparing sensory neurons (given the relatively intact proprioception) which raised the suspicion for APN; but given that this is a diagnosis of exclusion, other testing was required. Bloodwork and T4/TSH levels were performed to exclude hypothyroid and diabetic neuropathies and the relatively mild increase in CK was felt to be inconsistent with polymyositis, toxin-induced, or necrotizing myopathy. Thoracic radiographs were performed to exclude the possibility of either megaesophagus (which would have raised the index of suspicion for myasthenia) or intrathoracic neoplasia. Abdominal ultrasound was also performed to rule out abdominal neoplasia and complete the exclusion of paraneoplastic neuropathy (as far as possible). Tick envenomation signs vary in severity depending on the species of tick—*Dermacentor andersonii* and *Dermacentor variabilis*, found in North America, generally produce a less severe form of ascending LMN paralysis than *Ixodes holocyclus*, found in Australia (in northern states). The general evolution of signs with tick paralysis is much more acute than in this case, with ascending LMN paralysis affecting the hind limbs followed by the fore limbs (and frequently subsequent respiratory failure) occurring within 12–24 h. Similarly, snake envenomation in Australia produces severe and life-threatening abnormalities in addition to LMN weakness—most commonly a severe myopathy as the result of myotoxins (with CK levels in the tens of thousands or higher) and coagulopathy secondary to coagulopathic toxins. Of the common snake species in Australia, the copperhead is most likely to produce neuropathic signs. There was no history of exposure to snakes in this case and the evolution of her signs was too long to be the result of snake envenomation. There was also no history of exposure to rotten food that could be a potential source of botulinum toxin. We ruled out myasthenia gravis on the basis of the normal AChR antibody titer, the normal repetitive nerve stimulation test, and the lack of response to pyridostigmine treatment (Cuddon, 2002).

Case 5

Patient signalment

A 2-year-old female spayed Akita mix.

History

The dog was presented for a 4-day history of progressive, exercise-induced weakness. She was initially able to stand and walk unassisted for several steps before collapsing in the pelvic limbs. This progressed to difficulty rising and, if assisted, collapsing in both thoracic and pelvic limbs when fatigued. Additionally, regurgitation had been noted after meals for the last 24 h.

Physical examination

T: 38.6°C/101.5°F   P: 90 beats/min   R: 50 breaths/min

- **Weight:** 29.5 kg.
- **EENT:** Clear corneas, no abnormalities noted.
- **Lymph nodes:** Normal, no peripheral lymphadenopathy noted.
- **Oropharyngeal:** Pink mucous membranes, normal CRT, no masses seen.
- **Integument:** Euhydrated, no abnormalities identified.
- **Musculoskeletal:** No change in range of motion, no effusion noted.
- **Abdominal palpation:** Normal, soft, nonpainful, no masses or organomegaly noted.

- **Urogenital:** Grossly normal.
- **Respiratory:** No nasal discharge, no tracheal sensitivity, lungs clear.
- **Cardiac:** No murmur or arrhythmia.

Neurologic examination

- **Mentation:** BAR.
- **Cranial nerve exam:** No abnormalities noted.
- **Spinal reflexes:** Normal withdrawal reflexes and patellar reflexes in limbs.
- **Postural reactions:** Normal hopping and paw replacement in all limbs when proper support was provided.
- **Gait assessment:** Nonambulatory paraparesis. When assisted, she was able to walk several short choppy steps in all four limbs before collapsing in pelvic limbs, followed shortly thereafter by laying down in the thoracic limbs. After resting, she could repeat the same motion; however if she was asked to ambulate immediately after collapsing she was unable to rise (Video 6.4).
- **Spinal palpation:** No paraspinal pain noted, no evidence of pain on tail jack.
- **Cervical range of motion:** Within normal limits.
- **Other:** None.

Video 6.4. Video of Case 5 showing poorly ambulatory tetraparesis with exercise-induced collapse. (https://vimeo.com/696941183; video.cabi.org/EMBXL)

Neuroanatomic lesion localization practice sheet

Use this space below to work through NALL for Case 5. When you have finished, turn to the answer section on the following page to check your answers.

Abnormality	Possible NALL	Possible NALL	Possible NALL	Possible NALL	Possible NALL	Possible NALL

Discussion on neuroanatomic lesion localization

Abnormality	Possible NALL	Possible NALL	Possible NALL	Possible NALL	Possible NALL	Possible NALL
Tetraparesis	Forebrain/ prosencephalon	Brainstem	C1–C5 myelopathy	C6–T2 myelopathy	Peripheral neuropathy	Neuromuscular junction

Neuroanatomic lesion localization, Case 5: Neuromuscular

Tetraparesis without evidence of ataxia suggests a neuromuscular cause. It is important to remember that dogs and cats with spinal cord disease will almost always have a loss of proprioceptive testing before paresis, and certainly before profound paresis. By identifying a lack of ataxia in this dog, the NALL is automatically narrowed to the neuromuscular system. Within the neuromuscular system, the NALL can be further narrowed to a peripheral neuropathy, neuromuscular junctionopathy, or a myopathy. Animals with a peripheral neuropathy are expected to have reduced to absent reflexes in multiple locations; animals with neuromuscular junction disease are expected to have a complete loss of reflexes; and animals with a myopathy are expected to have normal reflexes—however with severe muscle atrophy or disease, reduced reflexes may sometimes be noted. In this case, normal reflexes would suggest a myopathy but there is one exception to this rule. Myasthenia gravis is a junctionopathy; however, it often presents without a loss of reflexes therefore making it indistinguishable from myopathic diseases.

Differential diagnoses

The differential diagnoses included myasthenia gravis (neuromuscular junction localization), immune-mediated and infectious myositis, and metabolic myopathy (hypokalemia).

Diagnostic testing and results

- **CBC:** No clinically significant abnormalities.
- **Chemistry panel:** Normal.
- **Thoracic radiographs:** Megaesophagus without evidence of aspiration pneumonia.
- **AChR antibody titer:** 1.6 nmol/l (normal serum titer, < 0.6 nmol/l).
- **Edrophonium trial:** An injection of edrophonium 0.1 mg/kg IV was administered and she was monitored for signs of improved strength (Video 6.5).

Video 6.5. Video of Case 5 after administration of edrophonium IV. The dog is able to more readily stand and walk unassisted before eventually collapsing in the pelvic limbs. (https://vimeo.com/696941306; video.cabi.org/PGDBN)

Case conclusion

The final diagnosis was acquired myasthenia gravis. Myasthenia gravis is an immune-mediated disorder caused by antibody blockage or destruction of the AChR. This is common in dogs and rare in cats (Khorzad *et al.*, 2011; Mignan *et al.*, 2020a). Three different forms have been described: focal, diffuse, and fulminant. The dog in this case had evidence of diffuse acquired myasthenia gravis due to the involvement of all four limbs' muscles and the esophageal muscles. Serum AChR antibody titers are the gold standard for obtaining a diagnosis of acquired myasthenia gravis; however approximately 2% of dogs will have a normal titer (Shelton, 2016).

The dog in this case was placed on oral pyridostigmine and assisted to eat through frequent, upright feeding. Monitoring for aspiration pneumonia is critical when managing patients with myasthenia gravis. The dog in this case was managed on pyridostigmine for 8 months, with monitoring of serum AChR antibody titers every 2–3 months. After 8 months the titer returned to the normal range, suggesting remission, and she was weaned off medication. No recurrence of signs was noted, and she was lost to follow-up after 5 years.

Case 6

Patient signalment

A 12-year-old female spayed domestic short-haired cat.

History

The cat was presented for a 2-month history of a left head tilt. She was noted to have effusion from the left ear when signs started and was treated with amoxicillin (dose unknown) for 14 days. Clinical improvement was initially noted, but signs relapsed after medications were discontinued. She is an indoor-only cat now, with a history of indoor–outdoor lifestyle over 5 years ago.

Physical examination

T: 37.4°C/99.4°F   P: 180 beats/min   R: 20 breaths/min

- **Weight:** 3.4 kg.
- **BCS:** 4/9.
- **EENT:** Mild waxy debris in both ear canals, remainder normal. No oral exam due to patient cooperation.
- **Lymph nodes:** Normal, no peripheral lymphadenopathy noted.
- **Oropharyngeal:** Pink mucous membranes, normal CRT, no masses seen.
- **Integument:** Dry, flaky skin.
- **Musculoskeletal:** Not evaluated.
- **Abdominal palpation:** Normal, soft, nonpainful, no masses or organomegaly noted.
- **Urogenital:** Grossly normal.
- **Respiratory:** No nasal discharge, no tracheal sensitivity, lungs clear.
- **Cardiac:** No murmur or arrythmia.

Neurologic examination

- **Mentation:** BAR, occasionally hissing.
- **Cranial nerve exam:** Left head tilt, positional rotary nystagmus, mild miosis OS, remainder normal.
- **Spinal reflexes:** Normal.
- **Postural reactions:** Normal tactile placing and hopping all limbs.
- **Gait assessment:** Ambulatory with mild vestibular ataxia and falling left.
- **Spinal palpation:** No paraspinal pain elicited on palpation.
- **Cervical range of motion:** Normal.
- **Other:** None.

Neuroanatomic lesion localization practice sheet

Use this space below to work through NALL for Case 6. When you have finished, turn to the answer section on the following page to check your answers.

Abnormality	Possible NALL	Possible NALL	Possible NALL	Possible NALL	Possible NALL	Possible NALL

Discussion on neuroanatomic lesion localization

Abnormality	Possible NALL	Possible NALL	Possible NALL	Possible NALL	Possible NALL	Possible NALL	Possible NALL
Left head tilt	Left CN VIII	Left medulla	Cerebellum				
Positional nystagmus	Left CN VIII	Left medulla	Cerebellum				
Miosis OS (reduced sympathetic function to eye)	Thalamus	Brainstem	C1–C5 myelopathy	C6–T2 myelopathy, or radiculopathy	Jugular groove	Bulla	CN V
Vestibular ataxia	CN VIII	Brainstem (medulla)	Cerebellum				

Neuroanatomic lesion localization, Case 6: Peripheral left CN VIII and reduced sympathetic function to the left eye

This cat has evidence of vestibular disease based on the presence of a head tilt and nystagmus. CN VIII are affected by loss of function of the peripheral nerve, brainstem, or cerebellum. To differentiate between these three localizations, it is important to evaluate the remaining neurologic examination for clues. Animals with brainstem disease will exhibit a loss of function of the UMNs and ascending proprioceptive pathways which is demonstrated as evidence of ipsilateral hemiparesis and reduced ipsilateral proprioceptive testing. Furthermore, reduced level of alertness (obtunded, coma, stupor) may be noted. If paresis, proprioceptive deficits, or reduced mentation are noted the lesion is most likely in the brainstem. Cerebellovestibular disease will manifest with signs of vestibular disease plus evidence of hypermetria, intention tremors, and/or truncal sway, suggestive of cerebellar disease. Absence of these findings suggests a peripheral CN VIII NALL. This cat does not have evidence of brainstem or cerebellar disease; therefore the signs were localized to the peripheral component of CN VIII.

Reduced sympathetic innervation to the eye may occur through damage to the sympathetic pathway. This pathway starts in the hypothalamus, courses caudally through the brainstem, cervical spinal cord, then exits the T1–T3 spinal cord segment, and travels cranially in the jugular groove to the cranial cervical ganglion. From the cranial cervical ganglion this pathway runs through the middle ear and along the trigeminal nerve to end in the periorbital muscles, third eyelid, and dilator muscle of the iris. Dysfunction anywhere along this pathway will result in miosis in dim light. The lesion in this case is likely in the region of the middle ear due to a lack of neurologic disease noted in the intracranial structures, spinal cord, or along CN V.

Differential diagnoses

The history and neurologic examination suggest otitis media/interna from bacterial or yeast infection is most likely. Other differential diagnoses considered include polyp with secondary infection or neoplasia.

Diagnostic testing and results

- **CBC:** Normal.
- **Serum biochemistry:** No significant abnormalities.
- **Thoracic radiographs:** Unremarkable.
- **MRI (brain):** On T2W imaging, hyperintense material is present in both bullae with ring enhancement on post-contrast T1W imaging. The brain was normal (Fig. 6.1).

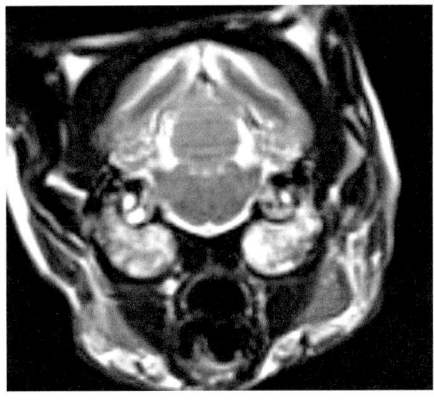

Fig. 6.1. T2W transverse image of the brain through the level of the bulla in Case 6. Hyperintense material is present in both bullae. Findings are consistent with otitis media.

Case conclusion

The MRI findings supported a diagnosis of otitis media, interna. A myringotomy was performed, including ear flush, culture, and cytology, on both ears. No growth was noted. The cat was placed on amoxicillin–clavulanic acid (19.5 mg/kg PO q12h) for 30 days and prednisolone (1.5 mg/kg PO q12h) for 3 days, then tapered. Clinical signs worsened after myringotomy but then improved 48 h later. The miosis resolved within 7 days; nystagmus and gait changes were absent at 30-day recheck. The head tilt remained present at the 30-day recheck which is often noted with vestibular injury in dogs and cats (Kent *et al.*, 2010; Rossmeisl, 2010).

The placement of this case in the current chapter ('Neuromuscular Disease') instead of Chapter 4 ('Intracranial Disease') may be confusing to some readers. This case placement is because the disease process affected the peripheral nerve, which is considered part of the neuromuscular system. In this case, the peripheral nerve happened to be a cranial nerve instead of a spinal nerve; however, the NALL is still the same: peripheral neuropathy.

Case 7

Patient signalment

A 2.5-year-old male castrated German Wirehaired Pointer.

History

The dog was obtained from a breeder as a puppy and has no previous significant medical history. Approximately 7 months prior to referral he began to have problems eating and drinking. He would pick up food normally, was able to chew, but would drop food into his water bowl. He was also noted to spend a long time drinking without lowering the level in the water bowl,

and frequently created a mess when eating. In addition, he was noted to eruc-
tate excessively and had been reported to have a history of intermittent regurgitation. Initial investigation and treatment by his regular veterinarian for GI
disease was unsuccessful. Serum biochemistry revealed an elevated CK level
(4000 IU/l; normal range, 75–300 IU/l) and no other changes. He was referred
to the neurology service for further investigation.

Physical examination

T: 39.6°C/103.8°F   P: 88 beats/min   R: 28 breaths/min

- **EENT:** Unremarkable.
- **Lymph nodes:** Unremarkable.
- **Oropharyngeal:** When prehending food the dog would drop food into his
  bowl and was very slow to drink from a water bowl.
- **Integument:** Unremarkable.
- **Musculoskeletal:** Significantly enlarged caudal thigh (semimembranosus/
  semitendinosus) and biceps femoris muscles, significantly enlarged triceps
  muscle. On palpation these muscle groups were obviously firmer and more
  fibrous than surrounding muscles.
- **Abdominal palpation:** Unremarkable.
- **Urogenital:** Unremarkable.
- **Respiratory:** Unremarkable.
- **Cardiac:** Unremarkable.

Neurologic examination

- **Mentation:** BAR.
- **Cranial nerve exam:** All cranial nerves were normal.
- **Spinal reflexes:** All spinal reflexes were normal.
- **Postural reactions:** Unremarkable.
- **Gait assessment:** The gait was nearly normal but on close inspection he
  displayed reduced stride length and a stiff limb movement in all four limbs
  (Video 6.6).
- **Spinal palpation:** Unremarkable.
- **Cervical range of motion:** Unremarkable.
- **Other:** None.

Video 6.6. Gait evaluation of Case 7 showing a short stride with stiff movement in all four limbs. (Video used with permission from Dr. Sam Long.) (https://vimeo.com/696941408; video. cabi.org/JCXOQ)

Neuroanatomic lesion localization practice sheet

Use this space below to work through NALL for Case 7. When you have finished, turn to the answer section on the following page to check your answers.

Abnormality	Possible NALL	Possible NALL	Possible NALL	Possible NALL	Possible NALL	Possible NALL

Discussion on neuroanatomic lesion localization

Abnormality	Possible NALL	Possible NALL	Possible NALL
Dysphagia/dropping food	Myopathic	CN V, VII, IX, X and/ or XII	Junctionopathy
Elevated CK level	Myopathy		
Abnormal muscle palpation (size and texture)	Myopathy		
Stiff gait	Myopathy	Peripheral neuropathy	Non-neurologic cause such as orthopedic

Neuroanatomic lesion localization, Case 7: Myopathy

Dysphagia as an isolated clinical sign can be a frustrating condition to investigate. CN V (trigeminal nerve) controls the muscles of mastication and dysfunction of this nerve can lead to dropped food, but most commonly this is in association with a dropped jaw wherein the patient is unable to close the jaw. On physical examination, the jaw hangs noticeably open and cannot be closed by the dog but can be closed by the examiner. CN IX and CN X (glossopharyngeal and vagus nerves) provide the sensory and motor input, respectively, to the pharynx and larynx. Dysfunction of these nerves may lead to difficulty swallowing. Localization to CN V, IX, or X did not accurately match the dog's clinical signs. CN XII (hypoglossal) dysfunction results in difficulty moving the tongue. Most cases of CN XII dysfunction have concurrent tongue muscle atrophy and may show deviation to one side of the mouth. This was not evident on inspection of the oral cavity. Dysphagia and difficulty prehending food can also be seen as a feature of neuromuscular weakness and has been reported in some myopathies (McAtee et al., 2018). Regurgitation may also be seen with canine myopathic disease because the canine esophagus contains a significant portion of skeletal muscle.

The gait assessment suggested a motor deficit, not a sensory deficit. The lack of reflex deficits and postural reaction abnormalities indicate the sensory nervous system is intact. Therefore, the spinal cord and brain are unlikely to be affected in this dog. Combining the findings on neurologic examination with the knowledge of the elevated CK resulted in a NALL of myopathy. Difficulty prehending food was due to poor muscle function.

Differential diagnoses

Muscle disease such as myasthenia gravis, muscular dystrophy, and infectious causes (T. gondii and N. caninum) were considered. Primary myopathies can be challenging to investigate. Although the full list of differential diagnoses is very large, many of these can be rapidly eliminated based on signalment and history.

For instance, centronuclear myopathy has only been reported in young Labradors (previously known as Type II Labrador) and Great Danes. Hypokalemic myopathy, hyperkalemic periodic paralysis, and Cushing's myopathy can be rapidly excluded based on bloodwork. Myotonic congenita, myositis ossificans, and episodic muscle hypertonicity present with quite specific clinical signs and can therefore be eliminated based on the neurologic examination alone.

Diagnostic testing and results

- **Serum biochemistry:** Albumin = 25 g/l (normal range, 27–38 g/l); ALT = 111 IU/l (normal range, 13–98 IU/l); AST = 143 IU/l (normal range, 17–84 IU/l); CK = 1826 IU/l (normal range, 73–522 IU/l).
- **Urinalysis:** Normal.
- **Urine culture:** No bacterial growth.
- **Thoracic radiographs:** Normal, no evidence of megaesophagus.
- **AChR antibody testing:** Normal.
- **EMG/Nerve conduction velocity:** On EMG testing, multiple regions with CRDs and myotonic discharges were identified—these were especially prominent in the gracilis and triceps muscles (Video 6.7). Nerve conduction of the sciatic and peroneal nerves was normal.
- **Muscle biopsy:** Chronic degenerative and regenerative myopathy that was most severe in the gracilis muscle and mild in the triceps muscle (Fig. 6.2).

Case conclusion

The dog was diagnosed with muscular dystrophy, with an unknown underlying genetic mutation. Muscular dystrophy is one of the most well-studied myopathies in dogs, in large part due to the fact that it offers a potentially useful model for

Video 6.7. Needle EMG of Case 7 showed multiple areas of CRDs and myotonic discharges. (Video used with permission from Dr. Sam Long.) (https://vimeo.com/696941557; video.cabi.org/QVMGF)

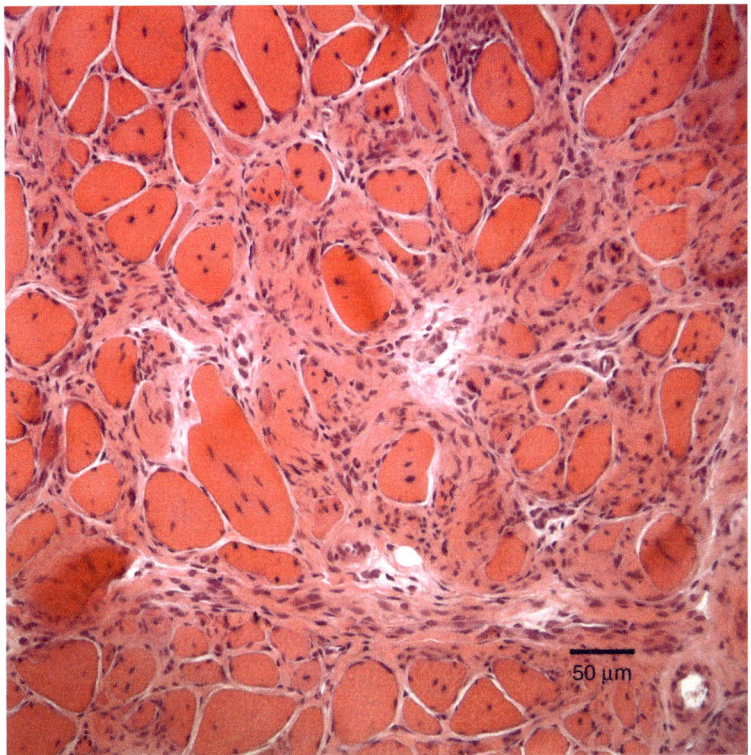

Fig. 6.2. A marked variability in myofiber size was present in the gracilis muscle of Case 7, with numerous atrophic fibers having a round to anguloid shape and of both fiber types. Scattered myofibers were undergoing splitting, numerous type 2C (regenerating) fibers were observed. Most myofibers contained multiple internal nuclei. Occasional necrotic fibers were undergoing phagocytosis. Endomysial and perimysial fibrosis were present regionally. These finding indicate chronic degenerative and regenerative myopathy. (Image used with permission from Dr. Sam Long.)

studying and treating muscular dystrophy in people. The most common of these is DMD—an X-linked, congenital myopathy. Absence of the dystrophin protein leads to contraction-induced microfissures which then disrupt calcium homeostasis, ultimately leading to cell death (Brinkmeyer-Langford and Kornegay, 2013).

Muscular dystrophy in dogs has also been reported as the result of mutations in the *dystrophin* gene, as well as with mutations in the *sarcoglycan* and *alpha-laminin* genes. The most well-known of the *dystrophin* mutations has been reported in the Golden Retriever, with X-linked GRMD providing a very close homolog of DMD in people. However, other mutations in the *dystrophin* gene have been reported in other breeds. In humans, at least 2898 mutations have been reported within the *dystrophin* gene. Unfortunately no specific treatment is available for muscular dystrophy, although gene therapy has shown some promising early signs of success.

The elevated ALT and AST levels were interpreted as being secondary to the breakdown of muscle as part of his underlying primary myopathy. The cause of the hypoalbuminemia was unknown—subsequent testing showed normal albumin levels. The dog was followed over the following 12 months and continued to live a normal life. Dietary modification, along with a food trial for consistency, managed his dysphagia. Exercise restriction was also recommended.

Case 8

Patient signalment

A 16-month-old female entire Mastiff.

History

The dog has been owned since 8 weeks of age and has no prior significant medical history. She presented for a history of weakness of 3 months' duration. Her owners initially noted weakness in her thoracic limbs. The dog was struggling to stand to eat and almost collapsing. She saw an orthopedic surgeon and radiographs of her fore limbs were performed which were normal. Her owners reported that she improved after the general anesthetic for the radiographs, but then her signs subsequently worsened. Trembling in the thoracic limbs was noted, followed by an unsteady gait in all four limbs, and then rapidly by an inability to walk on all four limbs. NSAIDs were prescribed which appeared to result in improvement to the point where she would repeatedly get up, walk 10 meters, and then collapse again. Vaccinations and worming were all up to date, and her diet consists of commercial dry food topped with raw chicken.

Physical examination

T: 38.7°C/101.6°F   P: 88 beats/m   R: 16 breaths/min

- **EENT:** Unremarkable.
- **Lymph nodes:** Unremarkable.
- **Oropharyngeal:** Unremarkable.
- **Integument:** Unremarkable.
- **Musculoskeletal:** Unremarkable.
- **Abdominal palpation:** Unremarkable.
- **Urogenital:** Unremarkable.
- **Respiratory:** Unremarkable.
- **Cardiac:** Unremarkable.

Neurologic examination

- **Mentation:** BAR.
- **Cranial nerve exam:** All cranial nerves were normal.

- **Spinal reflexes:** Normal to increased reflexes in the pelvic limbs with some evidence of clonus in patellar and cranial tibial reflexes; normal in both thoracic limbs.
- **Postural reactions:** Postural reactions were normal.
- **Gait assessment:** Due to the dog's size and weight gait assessment was difficult. The dog had nonambulatory tetraparesis. With assistance to rise she would take relatively normal steps with tremors in all four limbs. After 10 meters she would lie down. After a period of time, she would repeat this pattern. When walking, the range of movement in all four limbs was reduced with sliding to place the limbs (Video 6.8).
- **Spinal palpation:** Unremarkable.
- **Cervical range of motion:** Resistance to dorsiflexion.
- **Other:** None.

Video 6.8. Video assessment of Case 8 showing nonambulatory tetraparesis. With support, she was able to walk several steps before sitting down. (Video used with permission from Dr. Sam Long.) (https://vimeo.com/696941658; video.cabi.org/GQXHL)

Neuroanatomic lesion localization practice sheet

Use this space below to work through NALL for Case 8. When you have finished, turn to the answer section on the following page to check your answers.

Abnormality	Possible NALL	Possible NALL	Possible NALL	Possible NALL	Possible NALL	Possible NALL

Discussion on neuroanatomic lesion localization

Abnormality	Possible NALL	Possible NALL	Possible NALL	Possible NALL
Exercise intolerance	Generalized LMN	Neuromuscular junction	Generalized myopathy	
Tremors	Generalized LMN	Neuromuscular junction	Generalized myopathy	
Abnormal gait (weakness)	Generalized LMN	Neuromuscular junction	Generalized myopathy	
Resistance to cervical dorsiflexion	C1–C5	C6–T2	Intracranial	Non-neurologic orthopedic disease of shoulders

Neuroanatomic lesion localization, Case 8: Neuromuscular junction or myopathy

The clinical picture in this case appeared be most consistent with neuromuscular weakness. Weakness of all four limbs, in the absence of signs of ataxia, suggests neuromuscular disease. The tendency to stop and rest frequently after activity, along with the shuffling gait and the tremors in all four limbs associated with weight bearing are the strongest indicators of a neuromuscular weakness. All of her reflexes were normal; therefore a peripheral neuropathy was considered unlikely. A junctionopathy could also be ruled out based on the normal reflexes, however myasthenia gravis is one of the most frequently diagnosed junction-opathies and most reflexes are normal in most dogs with myasthenia gravis. Therefore, a myopathy or a junctionopathy was listed as the NALL for this case.

The dog's resistance to dorsiflexion of the cervical spine also raised the possibility of a separate problem within the cervical spine and given her breed we were unable to rule out a subtle cervical spondylomyelopathy in addition to her neuromuscular weakness. She did not have evidence of a myelopathy on examination.

Differential diagnoses

The differential diagnoses for the tetraparesis included myasthenia gravis (neu-romuscular junction localization), immune-mediated and infectious myositis.

Diagnostic testing and results

- **CBC/Biochemistry panel:** CK = 527 IU/l (range, 73–510 IU/l). Remainder unremarkable.
- **Orthopedic radiographs (stifles, hips, elbows bilaterally):** Unremarkable.

- **Thoracic radiographs:** Unremarkable.
- **MRI (cervical spine):** Unremarkable.
- **AChR antibody testing:** 2.82 nmol/l (normal, < 0.60 nmol/l).

Case conclusion

A diagnosis of myasthenia gravis was made based on the elevated AChR antibody titer. The elevated CK level was assumed to be the result of prolonged recumbency. The dog was started on pyridostigmine at a dose of 1 mg/kg PO q12h, and her owners reported she was able to walk unassisted within 1 week. This dose was continued for the following 12 months. A subsequent antibody titer, performed at her referring veterinarian at 12 months, was normal; therefore the pyridostigmine was discontinued.

Acquired myasthenia gravis results from an autoimmune attack against the neuromuscular junction. In the majority of cases in dogs this is due to the generation of autoantibodies against the AChR, but a small number of cases have been reported in which the antibodies target a different protein, muscle-specific protein kinase (Shelton *et al.*, 2001). The term myasthenia gravis is now only used to describe autoimmune attack on the neuromuscular junction and does not include causes of congenital myasthenia gravis.

Sadly, the prognosis for this condition overall remains guarded, with up to 40–60% of patients not surviving 12 months post diagnosis (Shelton and Lindstrom, 2001; Khorzad *et al.*, 2011). However, for those that do survive, long-term remission is relatively common, with a significant number of both dogs and cats achieving both clinical and immune remission (resolution of clinical signs and a return to seronegative AChR titers) (Shelton and Lindstrom, 2001; Mignan *et al.*, 2020b).

References

Brinkmeyer-Langford, C. and Kornegay, J. (2013) Comparative genomics of X-linked muscular dystrophies: the Golden Retriever model. *Current Genomics* 14(5), 330–342. doi: 10.2174/13892029113149990004.

Cuddon, P.A. (2002) Acquired canine peripheral neuropathies. *Veterinary Clinics of North America: Small Animal Practice* 32(1), 207–249. doi: 10.1016/S0195-5616(03)00086-X.

de Lahunta, A. and Glass, E. (2009) *Veterinary Neuroanatomy and Clinical Neurology*, 3rd edn. Saunders Elsevier, St. Louis, Missouri.

Evans, J., Levesque, D. and Shelton, G.D. (2004) Canine inflammatory myopathies: a clinico-pathologic review of 200 cases. *Journal of Veterinary Internal Medicine* 18(5), 679–691. doi: 10.1892/0891-6640(2004)18<679:CIMACR>2.0.CO;2.

Halstead, S.K., Gourlay, D.S., Penderis, J., Bianchi, E., Dondi, M., *et al.* (2022) Serum anti-GM2 and anti-GalNAc-GD1a IgG antibodies are biomarkers for acute canine polyradiculoneuritis. *Journal of Small Animal Practice* 63(2), 104–112. doi: 10.1111/jsap.13439.

Hankel, S., Shelton, G.D. and Engvall, E. (2006) Sarcolemma-specific autoantibodies in canine inflammatory myopathy. *Veterinary Immunology and Immunopathology* 113(1–2), 1–10. doi: 10.1016/j.vetimm.2006.03.025.

Kent, M., Platt, S.R. and Schatzberg, S.J. (2010) The neurology of balance: function and dysfunction of the vestibular system in dogs and cats. *Veterinary Journal* 185(3), 247–258. doi: 10.1016/j.tvjl.2009.10.029.

Khorzad, R., Whelan, M., Sisson, A. and Shelton, G.D. (2011) Myasthenia gravis in dogs with an emphasis on treatment and critical care management. *Journal of Veterinary Emergency and Critical Care* 21(3), 193–208. doi: 10.1111/j.1476-4431.2011.00636.x.

McAtee, B.B., Heseltine, J.C., Guo, L.T., Willard, M.D. and Shelton, G.D. (2018) Dysphagia and esophageal dysfunction due to dystrophin deficient muscular dystrophy in a male Spanish water spaniel. *Veterinary Quarterly* 38(1), 28–32. doi: 10.1080/01652176.2018.1435939.

Mignan, T., Targett, M. and Lowrie, M. (2020a) Classification of myasthenia gravis and congenital myasthenic syndromes in dogs and cats. *Journal of Veterinary Internal Medicine* 34(5), 1707–1717. doi: 10.1111/jvim.15855.

Mignan, T., Garosi, L., Targett, M. and Lowrie, M. (2020b) Long-term outcome of cats with acquired myasthenia gravis without evidence of a cranial mediastinal mass. *Journal of Veterinary Internal Medicine* 34(1), 247–252.

Rossmeisl, J.H. Jr (2010) Vestibular disease in dogs and cats. *Veterinary Clinics of North America: Small Animal Practice* 40(1), 81–100. doi: 10.1016/j.cvsm.2009.09.007.

Shelton, G.D. (2016) Myasthenia gravis and congenital myasthenic syndromes in dogs and cats: a history and mini-review. *Neuromuscular Disorders* 26(6), 331–334. doi: 10.1016/j.nmd.2016.03.002.

Shelton, G.D. and Lindstrom, J. (2001) Spontaneous remission in canine myasthenia gravis: implications for assessing human MG therapies. *Neurology* 57(11), 2139–2141.

Shelton, G.D., Skeie, G.O., Kass, P.H. and Aarli, J.A. (2001) Titin and ryanodine receptor autoantibodies in dogs with thymoma and late-onset myasthenia gravis. *Veterinary Immunology and Immunopathology* 78(1), 97–105. doi: 10.1016/S0165-2427(00)00255-5.

Skerritt, G.C. (2018) *Applied Anatomy of the Central Nervous System of Domestic Animals*, 2nd edn. Wiley, Hoboken, New Jersey.

7   Multifocal Disease

Heidi Barnes Heller[1]*, Julien Guevar[2]
and Devon Hague[3]

[1]Barnes Veterinary Specialty Services, Madison, Wisconsin, USA; [2]University
of Bern, Bern, Switzerland; [3]University of Illinois, Urbana, Illinois, USA

Unless otherwise noted, all images and videos are owned by the lead author.

Case 1

Patient signalment

An 8-year-old castrated male English Setter.

History

The patient was evaluated for an approximately 2-month history of progressive weakness and incoordination. His signs were first noted after running and slipping in the house, at which time his pelvic limbs splayed out from under him. Shortly thereafter, the patient began limping on his right pelvic limb and he was taken to his primary care veterinarian. Radiographs of his chest, lower spine, and pelvic limbs were taken, no abnormalities were noted. The dog was prescribed carprofen, gabapentin, and doxycycline (unknown doses and duration); progression was noted and attributed to the gabapentin, therefore it was discontinued. His signs continued to progress to include knuckling on his right pelvic limb and worsening incoordination.

Approximately 3 weeks prior to presentation, the carprofen and doxycycline were discontinued, and he was prescribed prednisone (dose unknown). In addition to prednisone, the dog was strictly confined until evaluation. Improvement was noted. The prednisone course was tapered and discontinued

*Email: barnes@barnesveterinaryservices.com

150   © CAB International 2022. *Small Animal Neuroanatomic Lesion Localization Practice Book*
(ed. H. Barnes Heller)
DOI:10.1079/9781789247947.0007

3 days prior to evaluation. Temporary improvement following chiropractic adjustments was noted, however progression to knuckling on the right thoracic and right pelvic limbs became evident 2 days prior to evaluation. Inappetence and neurologic progression prompted consultation with a neurologist.

Physical examination

T: 36.6°C/97.9°F   P: 72 beats/min   R: 20 breaths/min
(Unable to increase patient temperature despite external warming measures.)

- **EENT:** Corneas are clear, no ocular discharge, normal conjunctiva OU. No inflammation or exudate appreciated AU.
- **Lymph nodes:** Normal, no peripheral lymphadenopathy appreciated.
- **Oropharyngeal:** Pink mucous membranes, normal capillary refill. No masses seen. No significant dental disease or gingivitis.
- **Integument:** Clean and smooth hair coat with no skin lesions or ectoparasites.
- **Musculoskeletal:** No lameness, muscle atrophy, joint effusion, or pain on long bone manipulation.
- **Abdominal palpation:** Normal, soft, nonpainful, no masses or organomegaly appreciated.
- **Urogenital:** Grossly normal castrated male. Moderately distended, soft, and easily expressible bladder; intermittently dribbled urine during examination.
- **Respiratory:** No nasal discharge, stertor, stridor, or tracheal sensitivity. Normal bronchovesicular sounds bilaterally.
- **Cardiac:** No murmurs, sinus bradycardia, pulses strong and synchronous.

Neurologic examination

- **Mentation:** Obtunded.
- **Cranial nerve exam:** Resting and positional ventrolateral strabismus OD, otherwise intact.
- **Spinal reflexes:** Normal withdrawal reflex in the left thoracic limb, diminished withdrawal reflex in right thoracic limb (decreased at level of the tarsus). Normal withdrawal reflexes bilaterally in the pelvic limbs and increased patellar reflexes bilaterally. Intact cutaneous trunci and perineal reflexes.
- **Postural reactions:** Absent paw replacement test and hopping in the right limbs, delayed placing and hopping in the left limbs.
- **Gait assessment:** Ambulatory tetraparesis with moderate to marked proprioceptive ataxia when supported (right limbs worse than left limbs), characterized by being able to rise after multiple attempts—falls after attempting to take one or two steps.
- **Spinal palpation:** No discomfort elicited on calvarial or paraspinal palpation.
- **Cervical range of motion:** Normal.
- **Other:** None.

Neuroanatomic lesion localization practice sheet

Use this space below to work through NALL for Case 1. When you have finished, turn to the answer section on the following page to check your answers.

Abnormality	Possible NALL	Possible NALL	Possible NALL	Possible NALL	Possible NALL	Possible NALL

Discussion on lesion localization

Abnormality	Possible NALL	Possible NALL	Possible NALL	Possible NALL	Possible NALL	Possible NALL	Possible NALL
Dull/obtunded	Prosencephalon	Brainstem					
Ventrolateral strabismus OD	CN VIII	Medulla (brainstem)	Cerebellum				
Decreased withdrawal reflex in right thoracic limb	C6–T2 myelopathy	Peripheral neuropathy C6–T2	Neuromuscular junction	Muscle (with severe atrophy)			
Delayed to absent paw replacement and hopping in all four limbs	Bilateral prosencephalon, left more than right	Bilateral brainstem, right more than left	C1–C5 myelopathy	C6–T2 myelopathy	Peripheral neuropathy	Neuromuscular junction	
Ambulatory tetraparesis	Prosencephalon (rare)	Brainstem	C1–C5 myelopathy	C6–T2 myelopathy	Peripheral neuropathy	Neuromuscular junction	Myopathy
Proprioceptive ataxia in all four limbs	Prosencephalon	Brainstem	C1–C5 myelopathy				

Neuroanatomic lesion localization, Case 1: C6–T2 myelopathy, brainstem, and prosencephalon

The loss of the withdrawal reflex in the right thoracic limb can only be localized to the right thoracic neuromuscular system (the peripheral nerves of the brachial plexus and neuromuscular junction) or the spinal cord in the C6–T2 area. Loss of reflexes was not noted in any other limb, therefore neuromuscular NALL is unlikely. In addition, the loss of paw replacement in the right pelvic limb along with paresis of the right pelvic limb indicated damage to the long tracts of the right pelvic limb. This finding, combined with the loss of withdrawal reflex in the right thoracic limb, suggests a lesion is present in the spinal cord rather than the C6–T2 spinal nerves.

The brainstem is also affected in this case, resulting in positional strabismus and obtundation. The positional strabismus suggests damage to the vestibular system. Resting strabismus suggests damage to CN III, or the midbrain. Therefore, it cannot be determined if this patient's strabismus is originating from damage to CN III, or the vestibular system, or both. To determine if the damage to CN III and CN VIII are in the brainstem or peripheral nerves, we must evaluate: (i) the postural reactions; (ii) the level of alertness/awareness; (iii) UMN signs; and (iv) the involvement of other cranial nerves. Loss of postural reactions and the presence of obtundation would suggest a brainstem, rather than peripheral, lesion localization for these cranial nerves.

Finally, temperature regulation is part of the function of the rostral hypothalamus, a part of the prosencephalon. Disruption of temperature-regulating abilities can occur with damage to the hypothalamus or the hypothalamotegmental tracts (de Lahunta and Glass, 2009).

Diagnostic testing and results

- **CBC:** Low lymphocytes and low eosinophils, consistent with normal stress response; otherwise, no abnormalities.
- **Serum chemistry:** No clinically significant abnormalities.
- **Urinalysis (cystocentesis):** Unremarkable.
- **Total T4:** Within normal limits.
- **Canine SNAP 4Dx Plus panel:** Negative.
- **MRI (brain and cervical spinal cord):** Multifocal severe intra-axial and intramedullary lesions affecting the brain, cerebellum, pons, and cervical spine—consider infectious or noninfectious meningoencephalitis most likely. Neoplasia cannot be ruled out but is considered less likely.
- **CSF analysis (cisternal puncture):** TNCC = 2330 cells/µl (normal, < 5 cells/µl), RBC count = 80 cells/µl, total protein = 780.9 mg/dl (normal, < 25 mg/dl).

Interpretation in this case is marked neutrophilic and mononuclear pleocytosis. No evidence of infectious organisms or neoplastic cells is identified. Inflammation due to infectious and noninfectious causes should be considered.

Case conclusion

Multifocal NALL (brain, spinal cord), combined with the patchy findings in brain and spinal cord, and the pleocytosis on CSF analysis suggest an inflammatory or infectious etiology. Screening for infectious etiology was recommended based on the pleocytosis and was declined by the owners. Treatment was not pursued, and humane euthanasia was elected.

Inflammation of the brain and meninges is called meningoencephalitis. Inflammation of the spinal cord is called myelitis. This case was ultimately diagnosed with inflammation in the meninges, brain, and spinal cord, and is therefore termed meningoencephalomyelitis. Infectious and noninfectious inflammatory causes have been identified to cause meningoencephalomyelitis in dogs. The majority of cases are caused by a noninfectious, inflammatory cause that is suspected to be autoimmune in nature, however the triggers are unknown. Visualization of infectious etiology on CSF is often unrewarding, therefore screening for geographically appropriate infectious diseases is recommended for dogs diagnosed with meningoencephalomyelitis. If no infectious etiology is identified, treatment with immune suppression is typically recommended (Granger *et al.*, 2010; Coates and Jeffery, 2014).

Case 2

Patient signalment

An 11-year-old Retriever mix.

History

The patient began having seizures 3 weeks prior to evaluation. He was noticed to be uncoordinated when coming in from the back yard. When he came in the house, he developed minor head tremors and then fell over to his side with whole-body convulsions and vocalization, followed by a recovery period of about 15 min. Two additional seizures occurred the next day. Prior to the seizure onset, the patient had started showing weakness in his pelvic limbs in the preceding 2 months. One week after the seizure onset, four generalized seizures were observed. This seizure lasted 1 min with a 20 min postictal phase. A fifth seizure was noted on the week of presentation. Thoracic limb weakness became apparent 3 days prior to presentation. No additional abnormalities were noted at home.

On the day of presentation, two seizures were noted. The first was at home, the second in the car ride to the hospital. All seizures had a similar ictal duration, with variable (15–45 min) postictal phase.

Physical examination

T: 39.0°C/102.3°F   P: 140 beats/min   R: panting

- **EENT:** Corneas are clear, no ocular discharge, normal conjunctiva OU. No inflammation or exudate appreciated AU.
- **Lymph nodes:** Normal, no peripheral lymphadenopathy appreciated.
- **Oropharyngeal:** Pink mucous membranes, normal capillary refill. No masses seen. Mild halitosis and dental tartar. No gingivitis.
- **Integument:** A 3 cm round, soft, freely moveable mass was noted in the left axilla region and a small skin mass was noted near midline at the umbilicus. Clean and smooth hair coat with no ectoparasites.
- **Musculoskeletal:** No lameness, muscle atrophy, joint effusion, or pain on long bone manipulation.
- **Abdominal palpation:** Normal, soft, nonpainful, no masses or organomegaly appreciated.
- **Urogenital:** Grossly normal castrated male. Palpable urinary bladder and patient able to urinate on own with a steady stream.
- **Respiratory:** No nasal discharge, stertor, stridor, or tracheal sensitivity. Normal bronchovesicular sounds bilaterally.
- **Cardiac:** No murmurs, sinus bradycardia, pulses strong and synchronous.

Neurologic examination

- **Mentation:** Alert and appropriate.
- **Cranial nerve exam:** All cranial nerves were normal.
- **Spinal reflexes:** Decreased withdrawals in all four limbs. Decreased patellar and cranial tibial reflexes.
- **Postural reactions:** Normal placing responses in all four limbs, normal hopping in the thoracic limbs and slightly decreased in the pelvic limbs.
- **Gait assessment:** Mild to moderate ambulatory tetraparesis.
- **Spinal palpation:** No discomfort elicited on calvarial or paraspinal palpation.
- **Cervical range of motion:** Normal.
- **Other:** None.

Neuroanatomic lesion localization practice sheet

Use this space below to work through NALL for Case 2. When you have finished, turn to the answer section on the following page to check your answers.

Abnormality	Possible NALL	Possible NALL	Possible NALL	Possible NALL	Possible NALL	Possible NALL

Discussion on lesion localization

Abnormality	Possible NALL	Possible NALL	Possible NALL	Possible NALL	Possible NALL	Possible NALL	Possible NALL	Possible NALL
Seizures	Forebrain							
Decreased reflexes	C6–T2 AND L4–S3 myelopathy	Peripheral nerves	Neuromuscular junction	Severe myopathy (rare)				
Absent hopping in pelvic limbs	Neuromuscular junction	Peripheral nerve	L4–S3	T3–L3	C6–T2	C1–C5	Brainstem	Prosencephalon
Ambulatory tetraparesis	Prosencephalon	Brainstem	C1–C5	C6–T2	Peripheral neuropathy	Neuromuscular junction	Myopathy	

Neuroanatomic lesion localization, Case 2: Prosencephalon and neuromuscular disease

Reduced or absent reflexes indicate a lesion in either the spinal cord segment associated with the reflex, or the neuromuscular system. In this case, multiple limbs had evidence of reduced to absent reflexes which is more likely to be a result of neuromuscular NALL. Although multifocal spinal cord disease is possible, the lack of paw replacement deficits and lack of ataxia in all four limbs are more consistent with neuromuscular lesion localization. The neuromuscular system comprises peripheral nerve, neuromuscular junction, and muscle. Reduced or absent reflexes would be expected with a peripheral neuropathy or neuromuscular junctionopathy and uncommonly seen with myopathy. Severe muscle loss with contracture can give the appearance of a loss of reflexes but this is the exception, rather than the rule, with myopathies.

Seizures originate from the prosencephalon/forebrain in all cases, regardless of etiology. The combination of reflex deficits and seizures indicates a multifocal NALL.

Differential diagnoses

Causes of seizures for an older dog with neurologic deficits include neoplasia, meningoencephalitis, vascular event, and metabolic disease (hypoglycemia, hepatic dysfunction). Idiopathic epilepsy is possible but less likely due to the neurologic deficits and there is no history of toxin exposure or head trauma to suggest those etiologies.

Causes of a peripheral neuropathy include metabolic causes such as hypothyroidism, hypoglycemia, diabetes mellitus, electrolyte disturbance, paraneoplastic syndrome, neurodegenerative, and less likely neuritis.

Diagnostic testing and results

- **Blood glucose:** 38 mg/dl (reference, 68–104 mg/dl).
- **CBC:** No clinically significant findings.
- **Chemistry panel:** Severe hypoglycemia, with no other clinically significant findings.
- **Abdominal ultrasound:** Hypoechoic nodules present in the liver and spleen, enlargement of both adrenal glands, sludge in the gall bladder, no identifiable masses seen in the pancreas.
- **Cytological evaluation of liver nodules:** Metastatic neoplasia.

Case conclusion

Insulin-secreting tumors, such as insulinomas, are highly metastatic and can result in seizures secondary to hypoglycemia and a peripheral neuropathy due to a paraneoplastic syndrome (Goutal *et al.*, 2012). Treatment options including consultation with an oncologist, medication to increase insulin resistance (such as steroids), and anticonvulsant drugs if seizures do not resolve with glucose regulation. Prednisone and phenobarbital were started, and he showed decreased seizure activity and improved strength. One month after starting treatment, the patient represented in status epilepticus and humane euthanasia was elected, without necropsy.

Case 3

Patient signalment

A 1-year-old neutered male domestic short-haired cat.

History

The cat was found as an abandoned stray kitten with his littermates at a few months of age. When he was first obtained, he was uncoordinated while walking. Shortly thereafter, he developed head tremors while eating. After he was neutered, at about 3 months old, clinical signs progressed. The cat had a harder time walking and appeared weaker. Since then, he progressed to having trouble standing up when he is laying down and is unable to use the litterbox; frequent accidents are noted. While eating and drinking, the cat will demonstrate head tremors but is still successful with prehension and swallowing. He is up to date on vaccines and is an indoor-only cat. The cat's littermates are all healthy, but the status of the dam remains unknown.

Physical examination

T: 38.7°C/101.8°F   P: 200 beats/min   R: 36 breaths/min

- **EENT:** Corneas are clear, no ocular discharge, normal conjunctiva OU. No inflammation or exudate appreciated AU.
- **Lymph nodes:** Normal, no peripheral lymphadenopathy appreciated.
- **Oropharyngeal:** Pink mucous membranes, normal capillary refill. No masses seen. No significant dental disease or gingivitis.
- **Integument:** Clean and smooth hair coat with no ectoparasites.
- **Musculoskeletal:** No lameness, muscle atrophy, joint effusion, or pain on long bone manipulation.
- **Abdominal palpation:** Normal, soft, nonpainful, no masses or organomegaly appreciated.
- **Urogenital:** Grossly normal castrated male. Small palpable urinary bladder.

- **Respiratory:** No nasal discharge, stertor, stridor, or tracheal sensitivity. Normal bronchovesicular sounds bilaterally.
- **Cardiac:** No murmurs, sinus bradycardia, pulses strong and synchronous.

Neurologic examination

- **Mentation:** Alert and appropriate.
- **Cranial nerve exam:** All cranial nerves were normal.
- **Spinal reflexes:** Decreased withdrawal reflexes in all four limbs. Decreased patellar reflexes bilaterally and normal cranial tibial reflexes bilaterally.
- **Postural reactions:** Decreased hopping in the thoracic limbs and absent hopping in the pelvic limbs.
- **Gait assessment:** Weakly ambulatory tetraparesis more noted in pelvic limbs. The cat is unable to rise in pelvic limbs and remains plantigrade in pelvic limbs while walking. He can ambulate five to ten steps prior to falling into lateral recumbency with titubation when resting in a sitting position. Intention tremors are noted when offered water. Mild hypermetria in all limbs is noted when walking.
- **Spinal palpation:** No discomfort elicited on calvarial or paraspinal palpation.
- **Cervical range of motion:** Normal.
- **Other:** None.

Neuroanatomic lesion localization practice sheet

Use this space below to work through NALL for Case 3. When you have finished, turn to the answer section on the following page to check your answers.

Abnormality	Possible NALL	Possible NALL	Possible NALL	Possible NALL	Possible NALL	Possible NALL

Discussion on lesion localization

Abnormality	Possible NALL	Possible NALL	Possible NALL	Possible NALL	Possible NALL	Possible NALL	Possible NALL
Intention tremors and hypermetria	Cerebellum						
Ambulatory tetraparesis	Prosencephalon	Brainstem	C1–C5 myelopathy	C6–T2 myelopathy	Peripheral neuropathy	Neuromuscular junction	Myopathy
Decreased withdrawal reflexes	C6–T2 AND L4–S3 myelopathy	Peripheral neuropathy	Neuromuscular junction	Myopathy (rare)			
Decreased patellar reflexes bilaterally	L4–L6 myelopathy	Peripheral neuropathy (femoral nerves)	Neuromuscular junction	Myopathy (severe atrophy)			
Decreased hopping in thoracic limbs and absent hopping in pelvic limbs	Prosencephalon	Brainstem	C1–C5 myelopathy	C6–T2 myelopathy	Peripheral neuropathy	Neuromuscular junction	Myopathy

Neuroanatomic lesion localization, Case 3: Diffuse cerebellum and peripheral neuropathy

This cat has evidence of intention tremors and hypermetria which are localized to the cerebellum. Although gait deficits in the cervical spinal cord have been described as hypermetric, the combination of intention tremors and hypermetria is highly suggestive of a cerebellar lesion localization. With a cerebellar lesion localization, reduced spinal reflexes are not expected. The spinal reflexes are isolated to the cord segment associated with the cell bodies of the reflex in question, peripheral nerves, neuromuscular junction, or, in cases of severe muscle atrophy, myopathy. Within the neuromuscular system, the NALL can be further narrowed to a peripheral neuropathy. Animals with a peripheral neuropathy are expected to have reduced to absent reflexes in multiple locations; animals with neuromuscular junction disease are expected to have a complete loss of reflexes (except with myasthenia gravis); and animals with a myopathy are expected to have normal reflexes—however, with severe muscle atrophy, reduced reflexes may sometimes be noted. Based on the evidence of reduced to absent reflexes this cat most likely has a peripheral neuropathy as the cause of its neuromuscular disease. The reduced hopping is attributed to reduced neuronal function through the peripheral nerve as a result of the peripheral neuropathy.

Differential diagnoses

Multifocal neurologic disease affecting the CNS and PNS in a young animal is suggestive of a neurodegenerative disease such as a storage disorder. Other differential diagnoses may include an infectious etiology (*Toxoplasma gondii*, FIP, or fungal infection (blastomycoses, cryptococcus) in this region of the world) or multicentric neoplasia such as lymphoma.

Diagnostic testing and results

- **CBC:** No clinically significant findings.
- **Serum chemistry:** Mild hyperphosphatemia and hyperkalemia, but not clinically significant.
- *Toxoplasma* **IgG titer/IgM screen:** IgG and IgM negative.

Case conclusion

The lack of evidence of an infectious disease was suggestive of neoplasia or a neurodegenerative disease. Gangliosides was strongly considered based on the cat's presenting signs and neurologic progression (Sisó *et al.*, 2006; Hasegawa *et al.*, 2007). Cerebellar hypoplasia, although a common cause of hypermetria and intention tremors in young cats, was not consistent with the reflex deficits noted in this case.

Additional diagnostic testing such as an advanced metabolic screen for neurodegenerative disease, MRI of the brain and spinal cord, neuromuscular biopsy and electrodiagnostic testing, and CSF analysis were recommended and declined. The owner elected supportive measures such as additional assistance with litterbox placement, assisting to eat/drink, and close monitoring of the patient's hydration and caloric consumption. The cat remained static, without obvious progression, at 2 months after discharge from the hospital.

Case 4

Patient signalment

A 4-year-old spayed female mix-breed dog.

History

The dog was evaluated for a 1-day history of generalized weakness, which had progressed to flaccid tetraplegia. The owner also reported some difficulty breathing. The dog was treated with carprofen, maropitant, and enrofloxacin at the referring veterinarian prior to referral to a neurologist.

Physical examination

T: 38.7°C/101.6°F   P: 60 beats/min   R: 40 breaths/min

- **EENT:** Not evaluated.
- **Lymph nodes:** No abnormalities noted.
- **Oropharyngeal:** No abnormalities noted.
- **Integument:** No abnormalities noted.
- **Musculoskeletal:** No abnormalities noted.
- **Abdominal palpation:** Nonpainful, no organomegaly noted.
- **Urogenital:** Normal external evaluation.
- **Respiratory:** Abnormal respiratory pattern with insignificant thoracic movement during the inspiratory phase.
- **Cardiac:** Bradycardia, no arrythmia noted.

Neurologic examination

- **Mentation:** Alert.
- **Cranial nerve exam:** All cranial nerves were normal.
- **Spinal reflexes:** Decreased withdrawal reflex on all four legs, normal patellar reflex bilaterally, normal perineal reflex.

- **Postural reactions:** Proprioceptive positioning and hopping were absent on all four legs.
- **Gait assessment:** Tetraplegia.
- **Spinal palpation:** Painful on cervical palpation.
- **Cervical range of motion:** Reduced cervical range of motion with ventroflexion.
- **Other:** Deep pain was present on all four legs.

Neuroanatomic lesion localization practice sheet

Use this space below to work through NALL for Case 4. When you have finished, turn to the answer section on the following page to check your answers.

Abnormality	Possible NALL	Possible NALL	Possible NALL	Possible NALL	Possible NALL	Possible NALL

Discussion on lesion localization

Abnormality	Possible NALL	Possible NALL	Possible NALL	Possible NALL	Possible NALL	Possible NALL	Possible NALL
Tetraplegia	Prosencephalon (rare)	Brainstem (rare)	C1–C5 spinal cord	C6–T2 spinal cord	Peripheral nerve	Neuromuscular junction	
Decreased withdrawal reflex in all four limbs	C1–T2 AND L6–S3 spinal cord segments	Peripheral nerve	Neuromuscular junction				
Absent postural reactions in all limbs	Prosencephalon	Brainstem	C1–C5 myelopathy	C6–T2 myelopathy	Peripheral nerve	Neuromuscular junction	
Cervical pain on palpation and reduced cervical range of motion	Referred intracranial pain	C1–C5 myelopathy	C6–T2 myelopathy	Non-neurologic cause			

Neuroanatomic lesion localization, Case 4: C1–C5 myelopathy and peripheral neuropathy

Acute C1–C5 spinal cord localization with secondary spinal shock was considered for this patient due to the normal patellar reflexes. The acute and progressive nature of the disorder together with the presence of the patellar reflexes made C1–C5 spinal cord with spinal shock localization most likely for this patient. Neuromuscular lesion localization with a high likelihood of a peripheral neuropathy or neuromuscular junctionopathy based on the loss of withdrawal reflexes was also considered. Although conservation of the patellar reflexes with such disorders would be unusual, it could not be ruled out that those reflexes would diminish at a later stage in the disease progression.

The dog's difficulty breathing could have been to diaphragm muscle weakness secondary to a central (C5–C7 spinal cord lesion) or peripheral (phrenic nerve) lesion. Respiratory compromise from spinal cord injury results from disruption of the relay pathway from the brainstem respiratory centers to the intercostal and phrenic nerves. This disruption results in a failure of inspiration due to loss of diaphragm function and/or reduced intercostal contraction. Disruption of the phrenic nerve as part of a neuromuscular disease results in failure of diaphragm contraction during inspiration (Kube *et al.*, 2003).

Differential diagnoses

Rapidly progressing neuromuscular disease affecting all four limbs may be caused by idiopathic APN, botulism, coral snake envenomation, or tick paralysis. Differential diagnoses for acute cervical myelopathy included intervertebral disc disorder (Hansen type I; ANNPE; or acute, hydrated nucleus pulposus extrusion) and vascular etiologies (fibrocartilaginous embolism or hemorrhagic myelopathies) with secondary spinal shock.

Diagnostic testing and results

- **CBC:** No significant abnormalities.
- **Chemistry panel:** No significant abnormalities.
- **Coagulation profile:** No significant abnormalities.
- **Arterial blood gas:** Arterial blood gas analysis included PaO_2 of 77.0 mmHg (reference interval, 75–100 mmHg) and $PaCO_2$ of 37.6 mmHg (reference interval, 35–45 mmHg).
- **Thoracic radiographs:** Mild aerophagia, otherwise unremarkable.
- **MRI (spinal cord):** C3–C4 intervertebral disc extrusion with extensive extradural hemorrhage (Fig. 7.1).

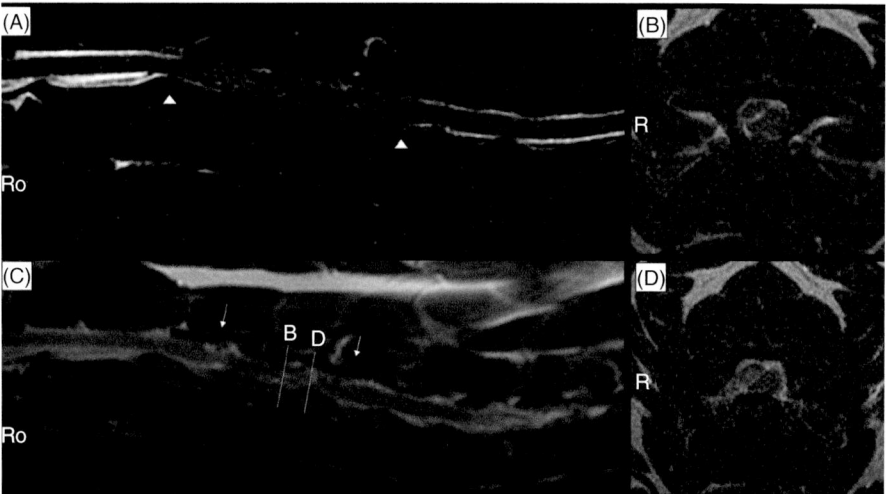

Fig. 7.1. In a midsagittal, single-shot, fast spin echo image of the cervical portion of the vertebral column in Case 4 (A), there is an extensive area devoid of signal from the CSF (arrowheads). In transverse T2W images (B and D), notice the focal extradural iso- to hypointense material compressing the spinal cord dorsolaterally at the level of the intervertebral disc space between C4 and C5. In a right parasagittal T2W image of the cervical portion of the vertebral column (C), there is a loss of the hyperintense CSF fluid and fat signal, along with the presence of multifocal punctate areas of hypointense material within the dorsolateral aspect of the vertebral canal (arrows). (Figures used with permission from Dr. Julien Guevar.)

Case conclusion

A dorsal cervical surgical decompression was performed. There was progressive improvement in the dog's neurologic condition. The withdrawal reflexes of the pelvic limbs returned to normal by the second day after decompressive surgery and the respiratory pattern improved after several days of oxygen supplementation.

Spinal shock is typically encountered after acute spinal injury in the thoracolumbar region; however, it can also occur with spinal cord lesion in the cervical spine. Experimental surgeries have shown that following transection of the spinal cord, the patellar reflex would disappear then return within 30 min to 2 h, whereas the flexor reflex may take between 2 days to 6 weeks to recover (Nacimiento and Noth, 1999; Ditunno *et al.*, 2004; Smith and Jeffery, 2005; Full *et al.*, 2016).

Case 5

Patient signalment

A 4-year-old, 24-kg, spayed female Bearded Collie.

History

The dog was presented for progressive tetraparesis. Six weeks prior to the consultation, the dog had acutely developed thoracolumbar hyperesthesia and an abnormal gait in the pelvic limbs that resolved with NSAID treatment. Sudden-onset nonambulatory tetraparesis had developed 24 h prior to admission. The pelvic limbs were markedly more affected with only mild voluntary movements. When provided with pelvic limb support, the dog could ambulate with a short thoracic limb stride. The dog had been admitted to the hospital at night, and by the following morning, the tetraparesis had worsened.

Physical examination

T: Did not assess   P: 100 beats/min   R: panting

- **EENT:** No abnormalities noted.
- **Lymph nodes:** Normal, no peripheral lymphadenopathy appreciated.
- **Oropharyngeal:** No abnormalities noted.
- **Integument:** No abnormalities noted.
- **Musculoskeletal:** No abnormalities noted; however a full orthopedic examination was not performed.
- **Abdominal palpation:** Normal, soft, nonpainful, no masses or organomegaly appreciated.
- **Urogenital:** Normal external genitalia.
- **Respiratory:** No abnormalities noted.
- **Cardiac:** No murmurs or arrhythmia noted.

Neurologic examination

- **Mentation:** Bright and alert.
- **Cranial nerve exam:** All cranial nerves were normal.
- **Spinal reflexes:** Withdrawal reflexes were decreased on all four legs; patellar reflexes were decreased bilaterally; perineal reflexes were decreased bilaterally.
- **Postural reactions:** Proprioceptive positioning and hopping were decreased on all four legs.
- **Gait assessment:** Nonambulatory tetraparesis.
- **Spinal palpation:** Pain on palpation over T13–L1 vertebrae.
- **Cervical range of motion:** There was no evidence of pain.
- **Other:** None.

Neuroanatomic lesion localization practice sheet

Use this space below to work through NALL for Case 5. When you have finished, turn to the answer section on the following page to check your answers.

Abnormality	Possible NALL	Possible NALL	Possible NALL	Possible NALL	Possible NALL	Possible NALL

Discussion on lesion localization

Abnormality	Possible NALL	Possible NALL	Possible NALL	Possible NALL	Possible NALL	Possible NALL	Possible NALL
Tetraparesis	Prosencephalon (rare)	Brainstem	C1–C5 myelopathy	C6–T2 myelopathy	Peripheral neuropathy	Neuromuscular junction	
Delayed paw replacement in all limbs	Prosencephalon (rare)	Brainstem	C1–C5 myelopathy	C6–T2 myelopathy	Peripheral neuropathy	Neuromuscular junction	
Decreased segmental spinal reflexes in thoracic and pelvic limbs and decreased perineal reflex	C6–T2 myelopathy AND L4–S3 myelopathy	Peripheral neuropathy	Neuromuscular junction				

Neuroanatomic lesion localization, Case 5: Multifocal spinal cord

Considered in combination with the history and progression, the deficits were best explained by a multifocal neurolocalization affecting multiple spinal cord segments. Although generalized peripheral nerve, neuromuscular junction, or muscle disease could potentially result in similar neurologic deficits, the absence of dysphonia and stridor (implying recurrent laryngeal nerve involvement), and the normal cranial nerve examination results, along with focal spinal hyperpathia were more suggestive of spinal cord disease. As with all multifocal NALL, the examiner may feel ill at ease when localizing to multifocal disease; however, at times, this is the most appropriate NALL.

Differential diagnoses

Focal spinal hyperpathia combined with a history of acute onset clinical signs suggests intervertebral disc disease (Hansen type I; ANNPE; or acute, hydrated nucleus pulposus extrusion) and vascular etiologies (fibrocartilaginous embolism or hemorrhagic myelopathies).

Diagnostic testing and results

- **CBC:** Severe thrombocytopenia (platelet count = 3×10^9 platelets/l; reference range, 200×10^9 to 500×10^9 platelets/l) and moderate anemia (hematocrit = 21%; reference range, 37–55%).
- **Coagulation panel (plasma concentrations of D-dimers, fibrinogen, and fibrin degradation products; prothrombin time; and activated partial thromboplastin time):** Normal.
- **Coomb's test:** Normal.
- **Infectious disease testing (*Ehrlichia* spp., *Anaplasma phagocytophilum*, and *Borrelia* spp.):** Normal.
- **Serum biochemistry:** No clinically significant abnormalities.
- **Thoracic radiographs and abdominal ultrasound:** Normal.
- **MRI (cervical and thoracic spine):** There were multifocal intradural, extramedullary and intramedullary lesions affecting the spinal cord and causing variable degrees of spinal cord compression and myelopathy. The various signal intensities were most compatible with multifocal bleeding (Barker *et al.*, 2015; Wang-Leandro *et al.*, 2017) (Fig. 7.2).

Case conclusion

On the basis of the diagnostic findings, a diagnosis of suspected immune-mediated thrombocytopenia with secondary spinal cord hemorrhage was made. Collection of a CSF sample was not performed because of the increased

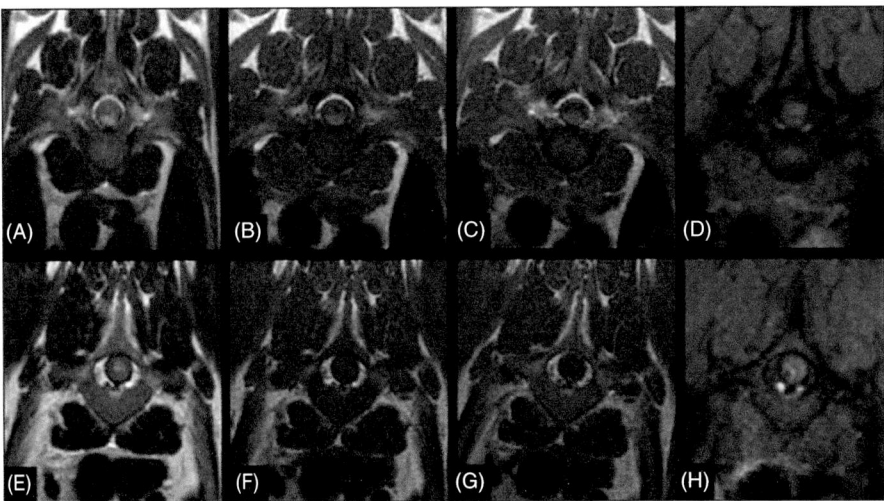

Fig. 7.2. Transverse MRI images of the thoracic vertebral column of Case 5. The upper row of images illustrates a ventral intradural, extramedullary lesion that is compressing the spinal cord. The lesion is hyperintense relative to unaffected normal spinal cord on T2W (A) and T1W (B) images and associated with mild peripheral enhancement after contrast agent administration on the T1W image (C); there is signal void on the T2*W image (D). The lower row of images illustrates an intramedullary lesion. The lesion is hyperintense relative to unaffected normal spinal cord on the T2W image (E), isointense on the T1W image (F), and there is no enhancement after contrast agent administration on the T1W image (G); there is signal void on the T2*W image (H). (Figures used with permission from Dr. Julien Guevar.)

risk of iatrogenic hemorrhage. Despite resolution of the thrombocytopenia within 48 h after starting immunosuppressive treatment (prednisolone and mycophenolate), little clinical improvement occurred, and the dog was euthanized.

Case 6

Patient signalment

An 8-year-old male castrated Golden Retriever.

History

The dog was presented for evaluation after a 4-month history of progressive mydriasis OS and a recent onset left head tilt. The dog did not have a significant travel history, was fully vaccinated, and did not have any medical concerns for which he was receiving treatment.

Physical examination

T: 37.8°C/100.2°F   P: 100 beats/min   R: panting

- **EENT:** Mydriasis OS, otherwise unremarkable.
- **Lymph nodes:** No abnormalities noted.
- **Oropharyngeal:** No abnormalities noted.
- **Integument:** No abnormalities noted.
- **Musculoskeletal:** Mild left temporalis muscle atrophy.
- **Abdominal palpation:** Nonpainful, no organomegaly noted.
- **Urogenital:** Normal external evaluation.
- **Respiratory:** No evidence of crackles, or wheezing.
- **Cardiac:** Normal rate and rhythm; no evidence of murmur.

Neurologic examination

- **Mentation:** BAR.
- **Cranial nerve exam:** A mild left head tilt was noted at rest along with absent direct and indirect PLR OS, mydriasis OS, mild left temporalis muscle atrophy, reduced physiologic nystagmus OS only, positional strabismus with absent doll's eye reflex (absent physiologic nystagmus when the head is tilted dorsally).
- **Spinal reflexes:** Normal spinal reflexes all limbs, normal perineal reflex.
- **Postural reactions:** Normal paw replacement placing in all four limbs.
- **Gait assessment:** Normal gait. No evidence of lameness, ataxia, or paresis.
- **Spinal palpation:** Nonpainful on palpation.
- **Cervical range of motion:** Normal.
- **Other:** None.

Neuroanatomic lesion localization practice sheet

Use this space below to work through NALL for Case 6. When you have finished, turn to the answer section on the following page to check your answers.

Abnormality	Possible NALL	Possible NALL	Possible NALL	Possible NALL	Possible NALL	Possible NALL	Possible NALL

Discussion on lesion localization

Abnormality	Possible NALL	Possible NALL	Possible NALL	Possible NALL	Possible NALL	Possible NALL
Mild left head tilt	CN VIII	Brainstem (left medulla)	Cerebellum			
Positional strabismus OS	CN VIII	Brainstem (left medulla)	Cerebellum			
Mydriasis with absent direct and indirect PLR OS	CN III	Brainstem (midbrain)				
Ophthalmoplegia OS in dorsiflexion	CN IV or VI	Brainstem (midbrain or medulla)				
Left temporalis muscle atrophy	CN V	Myopathy (temporalis muscle)				

Neuroanatomic lesion localization, Case 6: Peripheral CN III, IV, V, VI, and VIII

Differentiating central from peripheral cranial neuropathies requires assessment of the gait for evidence of a proprioceptive ataxia and ipsilateral hemiparesis, observation of a change in mentation, or observation of decreased postural reactions (ipsilateral or contralateral). Absence of these findings suggests a peripheral cranial neuropathy.

Identification of ophthalmoplegia (absent doll's eye reflex, absent physiologic nystagmus) is caused by a lesion affecting the innervation to the extraocular structures; specifically CN III, IV, and/or VI. Depending on the direction of the loss, one may be able to determine if the loss is specific to CN III, IV, or VI. Absent physiologic nystagmus when directing the eye medially (in the case of the left eye, it would be when the head is turned to the right) suggests damage to CN IV; absent nystagmus to the lateral direction suggests damage to CN III. In this case, a loss of physiologic nystagmus in both directions suggests damage to CN III and CN IV, however preservation of corneal retraction with the corneal reflex suggests CN VI may still be partially or fully intact.

The PLR pathway goes from CN II to the midbrain where it synapses on the parasympathetic nucleus of CN III and then travels along with CN III to the iris for pupillary constriction. In this case menace response was intact, therefore CN II was considered normal, and without a change in mentation, gait, or postural reactions the lesion causing absent PLR is likely to be peripheral CN III.

Lastly, the dog had evidence of a mild left head tilt and temporalis muscle atrophy. The head tilt is attributed to damage to CN VIII rather than brainstem due to the absence of paw replacement deficits, hemiparesis, or a change in mentation. The cerebellum is not affected because of a lack of hypermetria, intention tremor, or truncal sway observed in this case (de Lahunta and Glass, 2009). CN V innervates the muscles of mastication. With denervation, muscle atrophy occurs. Although a lesion in the muscles of mastication cannot be excluded based on the examination alone in this patient, the findings of multiple other cranial neuropathies lead the reviewer to consider damage to CN V more than a myopathy. Damage to CN III, IV, V, VI, and occasionally VIII can result from a lesion in the cavernous sinus. This localization was suspected in this case.

Differential diagnoses

Lesions of the cavernous sinus are most commonly neoplastic; however, a granuloma cannot be ruled out. Infectious etiology such as fungal disease or, less commonly, bacterial infection could be considered in addition to non-infectious, inflammatory granuloma.

Diagnostic tests

- **CBC:** Unremarkable.
- **Chemistry panel:** No significant abnormalities.

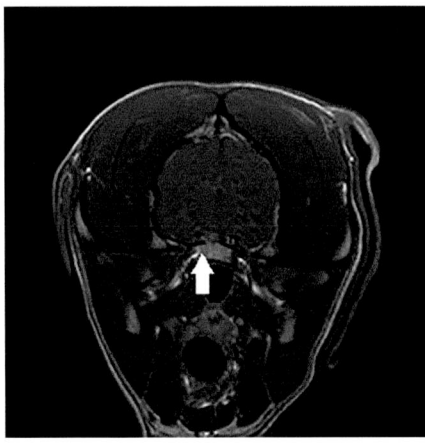

Fig. 7.3. T1W post-contrast transverse MRI at the level of the optic nerves. The mass is uniformly contrast enhancing, extra-axial and slightly right side of mid line (arrow) in the region of the right cavernous sinus.

- **Chest radiographs:** Normal.
- **Brain MRI:** On T2W imaging a hyperintense mass was noted at the level of the caudal left thalamus along the ventral aspect of the brain. The lesion was uniformly contrast-enhancing and consistent with neoplasia. The mass was located in the cavernous sinus and was most consistent with a meningioma (Fig. 7.3).
- **CSF (cisternal):** TNCC = 0; RBCs = 5 cells/µl (reference, < 0 cells/µl), total protein = 18 µg/ml (reference, < 25 µg/ml). No cytologic evidence of disease.

Case conclusion

Based on the findings, neoplasia was considered the most likely etiology and therefore radiation therapy was recommended. The dog was referred to a radiation oncologist and underwent definitive fractionated radiation therapy, being lost to follow-up 1 year later.

The cavernous sinus is a paired venous sinus that extends on either side of the pituitary gland on the ventral aspect of the skull. Lesions in the cavernous sinus may result in cavernous sinus syndrome, which is defined as deficits of more than one cranial nerve that traverses the sinus (Rossmeisl *et al.*, 2005; Jones *et al.*, 2018). CN III, IV, V, and VI course through this region to the eye and can be affected by a mass in this region. The most common clinical signs are ophthalmoplegia and mydriasis which are attributed to damage to CN III, IV, and VI.

Case 7

Patient signalment

An 8-year-old female spayed Doberman Pinscher.

History

The dog was presented for a 3-week history of progressive tetraparesis and low head carriage. She had a history of yelping when moving her neck approximately 1 year prior to presentation which was managed with an NSAID of unknown dose, and clinical signs were reported to improve. Over the past 6 months, the dog was noted to have a decrease of energy and a change in the tone of her bark. During the most recent 3 weeks, she was noted to stumble occasionally in the pelvic limbs. She had not sustained any known trauma and was up to date on all required vaccinations.

Physical examination

T: 38.7°C/101.6°F   P: 82 beats/min   R: 30 breaths/min

- **EENT:** No abnormalities.
- **Lymph nodes:** No abnormalities noted.
- **Oropharyngeal:** No abnormalities noted.
- **Integument:** Patchy alopecia over the bilateral flank.
- **Musculoskeletal:** No abnormalities noted.
- **Abdominal palpation:** Nonpainful, no organomegaly noted.
- **Urogenital:** Normal external evaluation.
- **Respiratory:** No crackles or wheezing noted.
- **Cardiac:** No abnormalities noted.

Neurologic examination

- **Mentation:** BAR.
- **Cranial nerve exam:** All cranial nerves were normal.
- **Spinal reflexes:** Reduced patellar reflexes in both pelvic limbs and a hoarse bark. All remaining reflexes were normal.
- **Postural reactions:** Absent paw replacement in both pelvic limbs, reduced to absent paw replacement in right thoracic limb, and normal paw replacement in left thoracic limb.
- **Gait assessment:** Ambulatory tetraparesis, more pronounced in the pelvic limbs, and mild proprioceptive ataxia in all limbs. No evidence of lameness.
- **Spinal palpation:** Mild discomfort with cervical palpation but otherwise nonpainful palpation.
- **Cervical range of motion:** Pain and reduced range of motion to the right and with dorsiflexion.
- **Other:** None.

Neuroanatomic lesion localization practice sheet

Use this space below to work through NALL for Case 7. When you have finished, turn to the answer section on the following page to check your answers.

Abnormality	Possible NALL	Possible NALL	Possible NALL	Possible NALL	Possible NALL	Possible NALL

Discussion on lesion localization

Abnormality	Possible NALL	Possible NALL	Possible NALL	Possible NALL	Possible NALL	Possible NALL	Possible NALL
Tetraparesis	Prosencephalon	Brainstem	C1–C5 myelopathy	C6–T2 myelopathy	Peripheral neuropathy	Neuromuscular junctionopathy	Myopathy
Proprioceptive ataxia in all limbs	Prosencephalon	Brainstem	C1–C5 myelopathy	C6–T2 myelopathy			
Decreased or absent paw replacement	Prosencephalon	Brainstem	C1–C5 myelopathy	C6–T2 myelopathy	Peripheral neuropathy	Neuromuscular junctionopathy	
Absent patellar reflexes	L4–L6 myelopathy	Peripheral neuropathy (femoral nerves)	Neuromuscular junction				
Hoarse bark	Brainstem (medulla)	Peripheral CN X or recurrent laryngeal nerve					
Cervical pain and reduced range of motion	Referred intracranial pain	C1–C5 myelopathy	C6–T2 myelopathy	Non-neurologic cause			

Neuroanatomic lesion localization, Case 7: C1–C5 myelopathy and peripheral neuropathy

The patellar reflex deficits indicate a lesion in the spinal cord at L4–L6, a peripheral nerve, or a neuromuscular junction. Without reflex deficits in any other limb, neuromuscular junctionopathy is unlikely. If the dog had a lesion at L4–L6, paw replacement deficits in the pelvic limbs, paraparesis, and pelvic limb proprioceptive ataxia could result. However, this lesion does not explain the gait deficits and paw replacement deficit of the thoracic limbs. Accounting for all the paw replacement deficits and gait deficits together would be a good starting point and therefore they should not be included when localizing the patellar reflex deficit. Therefore, the absent patellar reflexes in the pelvic limbs are most likely caused by a peripheral neuropathy affecting the femoral nerves. The recurrent laryngeal nerve is one of the longest nerves in the body and is commonly involved with peripheral neuropathic diseases. In this case, both the hoarse bark and the absent femoral reflexes could be explained by a peripheral neuropathy.

The second lesion would need to account for the paw replacement deficits, gait abnormalities, and cervical pain. Without evidence of intracranial disease (no history of seizures, change in mentation, and no cranial nerve deficits) the lesion is expected to be caudal to C1. Paw replacement deficits in three of four limbs, without thoracic limb reflex deficits, would indicate a lesion cranial to C5. Therefore, the second lesion is a C1–C5 myelopathy causing paw replacement deficits in three of four limbs, proprioceptive ataxia, tetraparesis, and cervical pain.

Differential diagnoses

A chronic, progressive cervical myelopathy in a Doberman Pinscher is likely secondary to disc-associated cervical spondylomyelopathy, but neoplasia and meningomyelitis cannot be ruled out.

A peripheral neuropathy in a middle-aged Doberman Pinscher may be secondary to hypothyroidism, diabetes mellitus, neurodegenerative peripheral neuropathy, paraneoplastic syndrome, or less likely neuritis.

Diagnostic testing and results

- **CBC:** Unremarkable.
- **Serum biochemistry:** Hypercholesterolemia, otherwise unremarkable.
- **T4:** 0.4 µg/dl (reference range, 1–4 µg/dl).
- **TSH:** 6.8 ng/ml (reference range, < 0.6 ng/ml).
- **Chest radiographs:** Mild cardiomegaly but no evidence of neoplasia or infectious disease.
- **Abdominal ultrasound:** No evidence of significant disease.

- **Spinal MRI:** Mild ventral compression at C4–C5, moderate ventral compression at C5–C6, and severe ventral compression at C6–C7 consistent with disc-associated (type II) myelopathy.

Case conclusion

The dog was diagnosed with disc-associated spondylomyelopathy and hypothyroidism (Bonelli *et al.*, 2021). Thyroid supplementation was started and follow-up T4 at the referring veterinary clinic was recommended in 30 days. Surgical and medical management for the disc herniations were discussed with the clients. Surgical management has a higher success rate for long-term improvement; however, it involves intensive postoperative management for client and dog as well as a significant financial investment. Medical management is less successful at providing long-term improvement, compared to surgery, but is a viable option for ambulatory dogs (Poad *et al.*, 2022). The owners elected medical management; therefore the dog was started on prednisone (0.5 mg/kg PO q12h) at a tapering protocol over 3–4 weeks, muscle relaxants, and physiotherapy. Additionally, the clients pursued acupuncture for added pain relief. On 1-month follow-up she was unchanged in neurologic examination except an absence of cervical pain and increased cervical range of motion.

Disc-associated spondylomyelopathy is commonly diagnosed in Doberman Pinschers. Common clinical signs include progressive tetraparesis, with proprioceptive ataxia in three or four of the limbs, with or without cervical pain. MRI is the diagnostic tool of choice; however CT and myelogram may also provide a diagnosis.

The underlying etiology of hypothyroid-induced peripheral neuropathy is unclear, however an effect to the Schwann cells or demyelination of the peripheral nerve is highly suspected (Suraniti *et al.*, 2008). Diagnosis should be made with a combination of T4 and TSH with additional testing such as for free T4 or thyroantibodies as indicated. Treatment with thyroid hormone replacement may not eliminate neurologic signs, therefore permanent deficits should be anticipated (Ferguson, 2007).

References

Barker, A., Williams, J.M., Chen, A., Bagley, R. and Jeffery, N.D. (2015) Suspected primary hematomyelia in 3 dogs. *Canadian Veterinary Journal* 56(3), 278–284.

Bonelli, M.d.A., da Costa, L.B.d.S.B.C. and da Costa, R.C. (2021) Magnetic resonance imaging and neurological findings in dogs with disc-associated cervical spondylomyelopathy: a case series. *BMC Veterinary Research* 17(1), 145. doi: 10.1186/s12917-021-02846-5.

Coates, J.R. and Jeffery, N.D. (2014) Perspectives on meningoencephalomyelitis of unknown origin. *Veterinary Clinics of North America: Small Animal Practice* 44(6), 1157–1185. doi: 10.1016/j.cvsm.2014.07.009.

de Lahunta, A. and Glass, E. (2009) *Veterinary Neuroanatomy and Clinical Neurology*, 3rd edn. Saunders Elsevier, St. Louis, Missouri.

Ditunno, J.F., Little, J.W., Tessler, A. and Burns, A.S. (2004) Spinal shock revisited: a four-phase model. *Spinal Cord* 42(7), 383–395.

Ferguson, D.C. (2007) Testing for hypothyroidism in dogs. *Veterinary Clinics of North America: Small Animal Practice* 37(4), 647–669. doi: 10.1016/j.cvsm.2007.05.015.

Full, A.M., Heller, H.L.B. and Mercier, M. (2016) Prevalence, clinical presentation, prognosis, and outcome of 17 dogs with spinal shock and acute thoracolumbar spinal cord disease. *Journal of Veterinary Emergency and Critical Care* 26(3), 412–418. doi: 10.1111/vec.12438.

Goutal, C.M., Brugmann, B.L. and Ryan, K.A. (2012) Insulinoma in dogs: a review. *Journal of the American Animal Hospital Association* 48(3), 151–163.

Granger, N., Smith, P.M. and Jeffery, N.D. (2010) Clinical findings and treatment of non-infectious meningoencephalomyelitis in dogs: a systematic review of 457 published cases from 1962 to 2008. *Veterinary Journal* 184(3), 290–297. doi: 10.1016/j.tvjl.2009.03.031.

Hasegawa, D., Yamato, O., Kobayashi, M., Fujita, M., Nakamura, S., *et al.* (2007) Clinical and molecular analysis of GM2 gangliosidosis in two apparent littermate kittens of the Japanese domestic cat. *Journal of Feline Medicine and Surgery* 9(3), 232–237. doi: 10.1016/j.jfms.2006.11.003.

Jones, A.M., Bentley, E. and Rylander, H. (2018) Cavernous sinus syndrome in dogs and cats: case series (2002–2015). *Open Veterinary Journal* 8(2), 186. doi: 10.4314/ovj.v8i2.12.

Kube, S., Owen, T. and Hanson, S. (2003) Severe respiratory compromise secondary to cervical disc herniation in two dogs. *Journal of the American Animal Hospital Association* 39(6), 513–517.

Nacimiento, W. and Noth, J. (1999) What, if anything, is spinal shock? *Archives of Neurology* 56(8), 1033–1035.

Poad, L., Smith, M. and De Decker, S. (2022) Comparing the clinical presentation and outcomes of dogs receiving medical or surgical treatment for osseous-associated cervical spondylomyelopathy. *Veterinary Record* 190(6), e831. doi: 10.1002/vetr.831.

Rossmeisl, J.H. Jr, Higgins, M.A., Inzana, K.D., Herring, I.P. and Grant, D.C. (2005) Bilateral cavernous sinus syndrome in dogs: 6 cases (1999–2004). *Journal of the American Veterinary Medical Association* 226(7), 1105–1111. doi: 10.2460/javma.2005.226.1105.

Sisó, S., Hanzlícek, D., Fluehmann, G., Kathmann, I., Tomek, A., *et al.* (2006) Neurodegenerative diseases in domestic animals: a comparative review. *Veterinary Journal* 171(1), 20–38. doi: 10.1016/j.tvjl.2004.08.015.

Smith, P. and Jeffery, N. (2005) Spinal shock – comparative aspects and clinical relevance. *Journal of Veterinary Internal Medicine* 19(6), 788–793.

Suraniti, A.P., Gilardoni, L.R., Rama Llal, M.G., Echevarría, M. and Marcondes, M. (2008) Hypothyroid associated polyneuropathy in dogs: report of six cases. *Brazilian Journal of Veterinary Research and Animal Science* 45(4), 284–288. doi: 10.11606/issn.1678-4456.bjvras.2008.26687.

Wang-Leandro, A., Huenerfauth, E.-I., Heissl, K. and Tipold, A. (2017) MRI findings of early-stage hyperacute hemorrhage causing extramedullary compression of the cervical spinal cord in a dog with suspected steroid-responsive meningitis-arteritis. *Frontiers in Veterinary Science* 4(SEP), 161. doi: 10.3389/fvets.2017.00161.

Appendix

This appendix contains additional blank Neuroanatomic lesion localization practice sheets for the reader's use.

DOI:10.1079/9781789247947.000a

Neuroanatomic Lesion Localization Practice Sheet

Use this space below to work through NALL for this case. When you have finished, turn to the answer section to check your answers.

Abnormality	Possible NALL	Possible NALL	Possible NALL	Possible NALL	Possible NALL	Possible NALL

Neuroanatomic Lesion Localization Practice Sheet

Use this space below to work through NALL for this case. When you have finished, turn to the answer section to check your answers.

Abnormality	Possible NALL	Possible NALL	Possible NALL	Possible NALL	Possible NALL	Possible NALL

Neuroanatomic Lesion Localization Practice Sheet

Use this space below to work through NALL for this case. When you have finished, turn to the answer section to check your answers.

Abnormality	Possible NALL	Possible NALL	Possible NALL	Possible NALL	Possible NALL	Possible NALL

Neuroanatomic Lesion Localization Practice Sheet

Use this space below to work through NALL for this case. When you have finished, turn to the answer section to check your answers.

Abnormality	Possible NALL	Possible NALL	Possible NALL	Possible NALL	Possible NALL	Possible NALL

Neuroanatomic Lesion Localization Practice Sheet

Use this space below to work through NALL for this case. When you have finished, turn to the answer section to check your answers.

Abnormality	Possible NALL	Possible NALL	Possible NALL	Possible NALL	Possible NALL	Possible NALL

Index

Note: The page numbers in italics and bold represents figures and tables respectively.

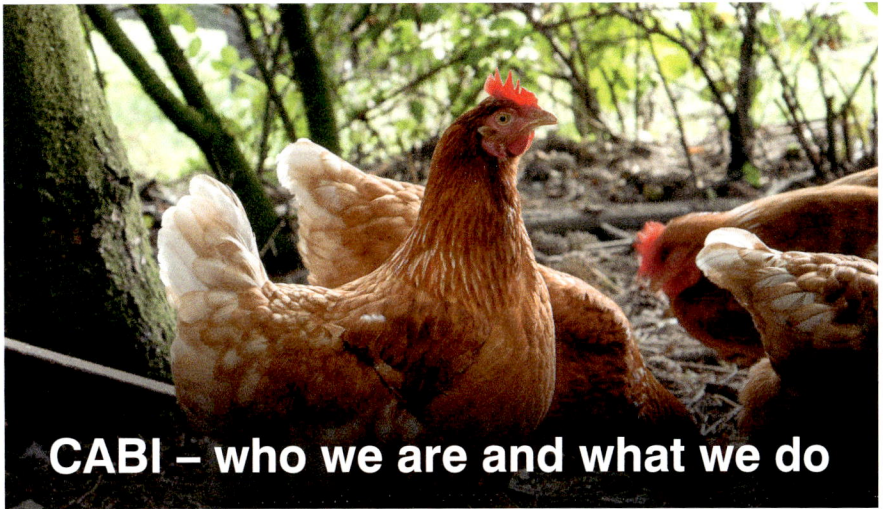

CABI – who we are and what we do

This book is published by **CABI**, an international not-for-profit organisation that improves people's lives worldwide by providing information and applying scientific expertise to solve problems in agriculture and the environment.

CABI is also a global publisher producing key scientific publications, including world renowned databases, as well as compendia, books, ebooks and full text electronic resources. We publish content in a wide range of subject areas including: agriculture and crop science / animal and veterinary sciences / ecology and conservation / environmental science / horticulture and plant sciences / human health, food science and nutrition / international development / leisure and tourism.

The profits from CABI's publishing activities enable us to work with farming communities around the world, supporting them as they battle with poor soil, invasive species and pests and diseases, to improve their livelihoods and help provide food for an ever growing population.

CABI is an international intergovernmental organisation, and we gratefully acknowledge the core financial support from our member countries (and lead agencies) including:

 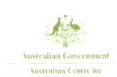 Ministry of Agriculture People's Republic of China   Australian Government Australian Centre for International Agricultural Research   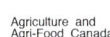 Agriculture and Agri-Food Canada   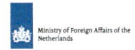 Ministry of Foreign Affairs of the Netherlands   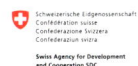 Schweizerische Eidgenossenschaft Confédération suisse Confederazione Svizzera Confederaziun svizra Swiss Agency for Development and Cooperation SDC

Discover more

To read more about CABI's work, please visit: **www.cabi.org**

Browse our books at: **www.cabi.org/bookshop**,
or explore our online products at: **www.cabi.org/publishing-products**

Interested in writing for CABI? Find our author guidelines here:
www.cabi.org/publishing-products/information-for-authors/